HISTORY OF
MENTAL HEALTH AND INDUSTRY
The Last Hundred Years

Volume X in the Series
Problems of Industrial Psychiatric Medicine
Series Editor: Sherman N. Kieffer, M.D.

HISTORY OF
MENTAL HEALTH AND INDUSTRY
The Last Hundred Years

Edited by

Pasquale A. Carone, M.D.
South Oaks Hospital
Amityville, New York

Sherman N. Kieffer, M.D.
State University of New York at Stony Brook
Stony Brook, New York

Stanley F. Yolles, M.D.
State University of New York at Stony Brook
Stony Brook, New York

Leonard W. Krinksy, Ph.D.
South Oaks Hospital
Amityville, New York

Library of Congress Cataloging in Publication Data
Main entry under title:

History of mental health in industry.
    (Problems of industrial psychiatric medicine,
ISSN 0277-4178 ; v. 10)
    Bibliography: p.
    Includes index.
    1. Industrial psychiatry—United States—History.
I. Carone, Pasquale A.   II. Series.   [DNLM: 1. Mental
health services—History—United States—Congresses.
2. Occupational medicine—History—United States—Con-
gresses.   3. Psychology, Industrial—History—United
States—Congresses.   W1 PR574M v. 10 / WA 11 AA1 H6 1982]
RC967.5.H57   1985   362.2   84-6567

ISBN 0-89885-207-2

CONTENTS

CONTRIBUTORS

HELEN M. ARNOLD, PH.D., R.N., C.S.
Associate Professor of Nursing
Adelphi University

WALTER E. BARTON, M.D.
Past Medical Director
American Psychiatric Association

Professor (Emeritus) of Psychiatry
Dartmouth Medical School

HENRY BRILL, M.D.
Clinical Professor of Psychiatry
Department of Psychiatry and Behavioral Science
School of Medicine
Health Sciences Center
State University of New York at Stony Brook

Honorary Consultant in Psychiatry
South Oaks Hospital

LEONARD W. KRINSKY, PH.D.
Administrator
Director of Psychological Services
South Oaks Hospital

ALAN A. MCLEAN, M.D.
Eastern Area Medical Director
IBM

Clinical Associate Professor of Psychiatry
Cornell University Medical College

STANLEY F. YOLLES, M.D.
Professor of Psychiatry
Department of Psychiatry and Behavioral Science
School of Medicine
Health Sciences Center
State University of New York at Stony Brook

PREFACE

On April 1 and 2, 1982, South Oaks Foundation, in conjunction with the Department of Psychiatry and Behavioral Science, at the State University of New York at Stony Brook, sponsored a conference entitled "Mental Health and Industry—A Historial Perspective: The Last 100 Years". The topic was timely as 1982 was the centennial celebration year of the founding of The Long Island Home, Ltd., parent organization of South Oaks Hospital and South Oaks Foundation. Our goal for this conference was to bring together individuals with expertise in various areas of the mental health field, individuals who could discuss the growth that has taken place in the past century.

In doing so, we have produced a volume that includes the history of the last century in the private hospital sector and in the public sector and the history of the involvement of the Federal government. We have sought and succeeded in presenting an overview. The nurse has been a truly vital part of psychiatric care over the centuries and we have a discussion of the role of psychiatric nursing in the past 100 years. Although the field of occupational mental health, as we know it, is relatively new, the presentation in this book gives an excellent account of the interdependence of mental health and industry over the years.

This present volume is a reflection of our continuing interest in the special problems and concerns of the mental health field with industry. The first conference in 1971 was entitled "Alcoholism in Industry," the second "Drug Abuse in Industry," and we have continued to sponsor yearly conferences in vital areas regarding the industrial worker and his family. Over the past several years we have discussed women in industry, special problems of retirement, and the equally important problems of the over-qualified or the under-qualified worker.

It is our hope that the reader of this volume will be enlightened as to the history of mental health in our nation over the past 100 years.

ACKNOWLEDGMENTS

It is usual practice in the preparation of a volume to give proper acknowledgments and appreciation to those who were actively involved in its preparation. In the case of this book, it would entail thanking the keynote speakers who gave freely of their time and expertise. The usual acknowledgment must certainly include the Board of Directors of South Oaks Hospital who have been actively supporting these annual conferences since 1971. Acknowledgments must certainly include our Executive Assistant, Catherine Martens, and our Director of Community Relations, Lynn Black.

We would be remiss, however, not to acknowledge those individuals, both known and unknown, who have lived over the past 100 years and who have provided the subject matter for this book. We would be equally remiss in not acknowledging the various mental health professional organizations which have provided leadership and structure during at least part of the past century. A hundred years of growth could not have taken place and this book could not have been written without an awareness and appreciation of all that has gone before.

Chapter 1

AN OVERVIEW OF THE LAST 100 YEARS

Henry Brill, M.D.*

The century which has now passed since South Oaks was opened has seen revolutionary changes in mental hospital psychiatry as well as in psychiatric practice generally. For a long period the story is virtually limited to hospital practice; other kinds of psychiatry are a relatively recent development. Looking back on the

*Dr. Brill has been in psychiatric practice for 50 years and has thus witnessed many of the changes described in his paper. Starting in 1932 at Pilgrim Psychiatric Center on Long Island, he was part of a large state mental hospital before the advent of the modern somatic therapies in 1937 and subsequently watched their development. Later, as director of the state hospital for epilepsy (1950–52), he observed the changes wrought by the use of modern anti-convulsants. From 1952 to 1964, at the state level he was involved with the introduction of the modern psychiatric drugs on a large scale and was able with R. Patton to document the state-wide revolutionary improvements in mental hospitals and subsequently publish a series of papers on the subject.

Dr. Brill has held such posts as First Deputy Commissioner of the State Department of Mental Hygiene, State Regional Director for Nassau-Suffolk, Director of Pilgrim Psychiatric Center, and Vice Chairman of the New York Narcotic Addiction Control Commission.

13

old hospitals, we find that some disorders which were once common have all but disappeared.

Some of the most distressing symptoms of patients in those hospitals have been so well controlled that it is hard to believe they once were major problems even a few decades ago. The recent development of non-hospital psychiatry and the spectacular new advances in scientific information about brain chemistry and the neurochemical changes associated with psychiatric disorder are all part of our history. What is perhaps most encouraging is that the technical advances have shown an acceleration in recent years and promise to make further important contributions to treatment in the foreseeable future.

This part of our story lends support to those who see all history as an account of endless advance, but there are other aspects that are less encouraging. The fact is that improvements in the mental health field have been quite uneven; some things have advanced rapidly, others more slowly, and in a few areas there has been relatively little gain. The entire story is of interest and has significance for the future; at least it provides some indication of what we may expect and it is, of course, of intrinsic interest in itself. We shall briefly examine some of these issues and try to draw some conclusions from this examination.

One area where we have made little progress has been the actual treatment of persons who are not responsive to the newer technologies. The treatment of psycho-geriatric cases, too, has lagged and so also has that of intoxicant abuse although there have been improvements in both. Another area of doubt has to do with public attitudes about psychiatric disorder. We try to persuade ourselves that we have improved public attitudes about the mentally ill—and this is undoubtedly true with respect to those whose symptoms have cleared—but where there are significant residuals or some active symptoms there is reason to doubt. I have in mind a family care program which had been in existence in Suffolk County for 30 or 40 years and which suddenly came under sharp attack during a recent period of loss of public confidence. I also have in mind some house burnings which occurred when a family care or hostel program had been announced for these buildings. Such things had not happened before in my experience on Long Island and may indicate that the public attitude is even less accepting of those with chronic mental symptoms or disabilities than it was when I entered this field 50 years ago.

On some issues there is room for real differences of opinion about the psychiatry of the past. At least some of this is due to our tendency to judge the past by the standards of the present. I was vividly reminded of this when giving a lecture to a group of mental health professionals and I described the use of malaria as a treatment for paresis. I was surprised at their response. They did not know what paresis was, so I described it with the more formal term of "psychosis due to syphilis of the central nervous system" but even then they were horrified at the idea of deliberately inoculating a person with malaria. Yet in 1927 this was considered such a significant advance that a Nobel Prize went to the man who developed the treatment; without it the disease was uniformly fatal in a year or two. Even more striking and well-known is the change of attitude about psychosurgery (lobotomy). In 1949 it was considered such an important advance that the originator was awarded half of a Nobel Prize. Today it is forbidden by law in some countries and is looked upon with horror by almost everyone. I said "almost everyone" because there are a few of us diehards who feel that psychosurgery did have a place, given the state of the art at that time, although it has been since replaced by medication. There are even some who feel that there is still a place, albeit a minor one, for limited psychosurgery in the treatment of certain cases refractory to all other methods. There is incidentally evidence that newer medications may still further restrict this use of the operation.

Keeping in mind the importance of the state of the art at a given time and the climate of public opinion, let us now consider the situation in 1882, the year that South Oaks Hospital opened. To begin with, it was a period of social pessimism. Social Darwinism was widely accepted by the intelligentsia; it was, incidentally, compounded of the work of several writers and Darwin had nothing to do with it. According to this idea only the fittest humans should be encouraged to survive. Mental disorder, mental defect, crime, alcoholism, and pauperism were linked and mental disorder was transmitted with increasing intensity to successive generations; thus eugenics was the order of the day. Thus the opening of a private hospital for mental disorder in 1882 would seem to have been counter to the spirit of the time. More specifically it was not long after the end of the period of psychiatric history which had been dominated by the "cult of curability" when hospitals vied with each other in publishing statistics which were manipulated to show up to 100 percent of "cures." The opposite view, "Once insane, always insane," became dominant and the nihilism of the late 1800's had a strong impact on psychiatry, and social services generally, for a long time. It may also be relevant to recall that the 1880's were a period of loss of confidence in government because of the scandals of the Grant administration and economic worries stemming from a series of financial disasters on Wall Street.

Let us go back now to get a closer view of what things were like in psychiatry in 1882. It comes from a book by Spitzka, published in 1883, which was the first systematic study of psychiatry in the United States since Benjamin

Rush published the first U.S. treatise in 1812. This was well before Kraepelin, and the terminology is a mixture of items drawn from French, English, and German psychiatry. It abounds in strange terms like monomania, transitory frenzies, primary dementia, secondary dementia, and terminal dementia.

More impressive than the strange terminology is the lack of knowledge which today is taken for granted. For example, Spitzka repeated the idea which was common at the time that "general paralysis of the insane," which he described quite accurately, was a multifactorial disease in which syphilis might play a role. It was not until later that the disease was identified as syphilitic in nature; the spinal tap was yet to be introduced into clinical practice, that was to come in 1890; the Wasserman test was not to be available until 1906, and the 1897 paper by Krafft-Ebing was yet to appear. He reported that a paretic inoculated with syphilitic material was immune to the second infection, proving that he already had the disease. Even in 1897, in Germany, this was so bold an experiment that it was published anonymously.

The pharmacological treatment of the 1880's was limited to sedatives and a variety of other drugs which have since passed from the scene. Spitzka makes the comment that the most useful general treatment was opium, a drug which had been used for psychiatric disorder for at least 2,000 years. Bromides and chloral hydrate were widely used also, and paraldehyde had just been introduced. In 1882 psychodynamics was still to come and at that time Freud himself was working with cocaine; his first book on psychological methods was not to come until 1893 when he published with Breuer. Only milieu therapy and moral therapy were available for treatment in the modern sense and they were widely used in hospitals of the South Oaks type.

Looking back on things, psychiatry was in a rather primitive state, and yet it *had* advanced over the previous 100 years. The sedatives were a useful innovation, all new with the exception of opium. Bleeding and purging had been dropped, and moral and milieu therapy had been established so firmly that they still remain a part of hospital treatment under various names and in various derivative forms.

If we are in a better position today than they were at that time, it is due to the work of those who went before us; this is underlined in a book by Kraepelin published in 1917 to describe the previous 100 years of psychiatry. It is written from the point of view of a university hospital and not entirely comparable to that of Spitzka whose experience was largely that of a consultant in a state hospital in New York. Today Kraepelin is often portrayed as the embodiment of everything that was wrong with the older psychiatry, but his actual writings convey an entirely different impression. True, the technology of his day was still primitive by current standards, but the man must of course be judged by the state of the art of his time. The quality of life which he sought to establish for his patients and his interpretation of what he saw was well ahead of his time. He pointed out that regressive behavior, often seen as a simple outcome of mental disorder, was in reality an artifact, either entirely or to a large extent. He called for a rigorous evaluation of the so-called medicines which had hitherto been used, and in questioning the effectiveness of the older methods, he helped open the way for the development of newer ones. In his call for more rigorous evaluations he was almost 20 years ahead of his time because it was not until 1935 that Bradford Hill introduced the controlled clinical trial which is the basis of pharmacological work today.

Kraepelin's critics may also be surprised to know that in his book on psychiatric history he insisted that seclusion could be given up almost entirely in mental hospitals; in his own facility it had not been used for 20 years with a single exception. He favored giving patients a maximum degree of freedom which was feasible and pointed out that family care, when it is practical, is superior to hospital care. Thus speaking generally, we find him advocating items relating to the quality of life for the mentally ill which are quite modern in their nature. He did point out that there were people for whom psychiatry had no effective treatment and this was mentioned as a problem for future research; unsolved in his time and still unsolved today although to a lesser extent than it was in 1923.

Another source of information on the last hundred years in hospital psychiatry comes in the form of official governmental reports, and we must recall that until after World War II there was virtually no psychiatry outside of mental hospitals of various types except a small amount of private practice. The quality of life in public mental hospitals is, for example, reflected in a 1923 publication by the U.S. Department of Commerce entitled, "Patients in Hospitals for Mental Disease." The national per capita annual expenditure for such hospitals was $282. In New York it was a little higher, $334. The state hospital population of New York was about 40,000 and the staff numbered some 6,800. For the U.S. as a whole the hospitals had some 225,000 patients and 34,000 personnel. Even allowing for the fact that the ward personnel worked a 12-hour day, the staffing ratio seems unbelievably low; today it is about six times as high, and the per capita cost is about 10 times as high. These figures by themselves tell a vivid story about the quality of life in these hospitals during the earlier part of this century.

Another aspect of psychiatric history, and a far more agreeable one, shows up in the figures for mental hospital population. Pellagra, which is today unknown as an admission diagnosis, accounted for 507 cases in 1923. It was estimated that the number of persons who had psychiatric disorder with pellagra in the U.S. was six to eight times as high; this is interesting in view of the fact that the disease was unknown in this country before 1900. More important, numerically at least, were the admissions of patients with syphilis of the central nervous system. They numbered about 9,000 or about 10 percent of all admissions and their hospital life was short. Today this disease has almost completely disappeared from our statistics, as has pellagra, and when a case does show up it is a clinical rarity. Similarly, there were 9,000 patients admitted to U.S. mental hospitals with psychosis associated with epilepsy, and this diagnosis, too, has virtually disappeared. These changes in statistics represent real advances in the technology of treatment. In all three cases a single effective medication had been found. And of course with this advance came prevention, primary or secondary. As is usually the case, other and improved methods followed and all this was so successful that the whole story has been generally forgotten, as has been the fact that until the early 1940's, most states maintained a hospital for non-psychotic, or normal epileptics, who required care because of the uncontrolled nature of their seizures. These too are now but an entry in the old statistics.

We now come to 1932 when I came on the psychiatric scene. Things were not much better than they were in 1917 or 1923. We used virtually the same drugs except that barbiturates had been added, but disturbed and regressive behavior was a major problem. Seclusion and restraint were widely used; about 40 per 1,000 patients were in one or the other at any given moment. Today there may be one or none. Hydrotherapy was the most advanced way of treating disturbed behavior. It was costly in terms of personnel and of limited effect; also it could be dangerous. With the coming of World War II hydrotherapy disappeared from our armamentarium simply because of lack of personnel. But the method was so deeply ingrained in the administrative structure that as late as 1955 these costly installations continued to be included in new construction. And, even then in the case of a new building on Ward's Island in New York, there was a vigorous debate before the actual tubs and controls were left out, but the pipes and tiles were still included, "in case we change our minds." Later these rooms were put to good use for milieu therapy.

Perhaps the most distressing and spectacular aspect of mental hospital operation which I saw from 1932 onward was the growth of resident population. This had doubled every 25 years since 1900 and was to continue at the same rate until 1955. In 1932 alone, partly because of the economic depression, the census jumped by 6 percent and that year the private mental hospitals actually lost population because of the same reason. For a while, we wondered whether private hospitals would be able to survive the economic storm; today they are more important than ever.

There were many other problems in the under-financed, under-staffed and overcrowded state mental hospitals of the 1930's. Tuberculosis was widespread and the crude death rate was some 20 times that of the general population in New York State in 1932. Even as late as 1941 an X-ray survey showed that some 4 percent of the patients had active tuberculosis. Deaths from psychotic exhaustion were not infrequent especially during the summer months and the "back wards" were filled with noisy, destructive, denudative, or assaultive patients, and wetting and soiling was a major problem. Even so, the improvement which had been achieved in public health measures was apparent in that the old typhoid epidemics were gone and so also the notorious epidemics of ersypelas described in the older literature. There had been progress but it was agonizingly slow. Occupational and recreational therapy were actively supported, but many patients could not be reached; psychodynamics was discussed but it did not exist as a treatment modality except in private practice which was on a small scale; outpatient services were limited in New York State to aftercare clinics and child guidance if one excepts a few pioneering academic undertakings.

One often hears negative things about the personnel of the mental hospitals in those days, but I can testify to the dedication and efforts of the vast majority of them. It was the bottom of the Great Depression and the recruitment situation was better than I have ever seen it since. Yet the simple fact was that the hospitals had been overwhelmed by the vast increases in census. In 1880 about when our paper begins the story, there were 81 persons per 100,000 in U.S. mental hospitals; by 1923 it had jumped to 245 and by 1955 it had gone—in New York and several other states—to some 600 per 100,000, and there were some areas of New York City where more than 1 percent of the population were in the state hospitals. Most troublesome was the fact that until 1955, the population continued to increase by some 2,000 per year in New York State alone. It was obvious that something other than hospital services would have to be developed to meet the vast need.

In 1944 the American Psychiatric Association published a centennial volume which reflects the slow growth of basic knowledge in the field but gives no inkling of the changes that were to come within a decade or two. There is brief mention of the shock therapies which had been in use since the 1930's and there was considerable discussion about the growth of psychiatry outside of the state mental hospitals, but the impression one gets from it is that the light to be seen was at the end of a very long tunnel. Yet the fact was that we were on the threshold of revolutionary changes in the mental health services.

Let us now take a few moments to see how the ground was prepared for this change because it did not come out of the blue. To begin with, there was a steady growth of evidence that mental disease, to paraphrase Hippocrates, was a disease (or a group of diseases) like all others with its causes and its cures. We had seen pellagra disappear once the work of Goldberger and others had been applied, although I still recall seeing cases of alcoholic pellagra coming to Pilgrim State Hospital just before World War II. Paresis had become a treatable and preventable condition with the appearance of penicillin. We had seen psychosis due to epilepsy virtually disappear with the introduction of effective anti-convulsants. And, in spite of all the doubts and reservations that were and still are expressed, it was clear to many of us that the major psychiatric disorders— schizophrenia and the affective disorders—were also responsive to somatic therapies even though they were "functional" in nature. Up until the introduction of insulin shock treatment in the mid-1930's, the mental disorders which had become treatable were all "organic" in nature, they had a known physical cause and thus a physical treatment was reasonably to be expected. The major psychoses which filled the state mental hospitals did not, however, have a known physical cause and it was a breakthrough of theoretical interest that some of these cases could respond to a physical treatment even though the bulk of them still did not.

There were still other indications of the link between psychiatric disorder and somatic illness. One of the most spectacular was a disease that came and went so rapidly that it has been all but forgotten. I refer to encephalitis lethargica. It appeared in 1917 and spread in a worldwide pandemic. Before it faded out in the late 1930's it had brought many thousands to mental hospitals with a bizarre combination of neurological and psychiatric symptoms. Outstanding was the associated conduct disorder which was perhaps the most severe that I have ever witnessed in any type of psychiatric entity and the behavior often preceded the neurological signs by months or years leaving one to wonder how many other cases of intractable conduct disorder might be due to a similar cause of lesser intensity. Interestingly enough the neurological residuals bore a close resemblance to the neurological signs associated with modern tranquilizer therapy including Parkinsonism and oculogyric crises. The neurochemical significance of this coincidence is only now beginning to be understood.

By the 1950's it had become clear that something more was needed to deal with public mental health problems. The experience of two world wars had left a deep impact on government awareness of the scope of the need, and experience with the second war had set the stage for social engineering in this field. The British experience too was an example of what might be accomplished in the way of social psychiatric approaches with emphasis on liberalizing mental hospital operations and utilizing community psychiatry. By a coincidence, the U.S. passed a Mental Health Study Act in 1955, the year that a new medication was introduced on a large scale for the treatment of schizophrenia. This proved to be a decisive year in psychiatric history. The mental hospital population in New York and nationwide stopped increasing and began a decrease that has since continued. In 1963 the Federal government formally entered the mental health field and community mental health services became a reality on a vast scale during the next few years.

Now, for the first time, the application of psychodynamic principles could be applied on a large scale in outpatient settings. Today some 4 million persons are treated annually for psychiatric problems and only a small minority come to any type of psychiatric hospital. It is not possible to show how much each of the various factors contributed to the revolution in psychiatric services that has gone so far to solve a problem which only a few years ago seemed to defy every effort. The advances in medical technology

in the form of major tranquilizers and anti-depressants undoubtedly played a major role and the impact on the operations of the large mental hospitals was immediate.
Within a space of months the wards became more quiet and
within a somewhat longer time other conduct disorders di-
minished spectacularly. Equally impressive was the sudden
cessation of the long-time annual increases in hospital census. Yet this was only part of the story. With the new mental health initiative on the Federal level, outpatient services
expanded and now psychodynamically-oriented therapy became available for the first time to hundreds of thousands.
The population decrease of the mental hospitals was accelerated by new laws and policies as outpatient treatment
with the new medications was established.

The basic aims of the community mental health movement had been achieved to a degree which no one had ever
dared to hope would happen in so short a time. But there
still remain those for whom we really do not know what to
do, as Kraepelin said, and many others who are not being
reached for a variety of reasons. The public and industry
are willing to accept back those who have been ill and have
recovered. Leaves are granted for mental illness as for other
types of sickness and there is third-party funding for those
who need brief hospital care and treatment, but for the person with chronic long-term disability, who has not responded to therapy, our situation is not much better than it was
in the time of Kraepelin.

State and Federal as well as local funding have vastly
increased and have eased the problems considerably of those
with long-term disability, but they still wait for further advances in scientific technology. Many of them are now in
the community, many more than before 1955, but there are
abundant indications that public attitudes about them have
not improved to the degree that some of us would like to
think; educating the public in this area, as in so many others,

has proved to be a far more difficult task than might have been expected, and sometimes it appears that ground has actually been lost. This is particularly true when psychiatric disorder is marked by violence and appears in the criminal courts. Regardless of how one feels about the academic issues in this area, it is easy to draw a parallel between the public reaction to the Hinckley case in 1982 and the public reaction to McNaughton in 1843; he was acquitted of a political assassination but left a controversy that still is unsettled in spite of the famous "Rules" that were promulgated to mollify the public. (Careful researchers have even been unable to decide on the correct spelling of his name often written M'Naghten.)

The abuse of intoxicants remains another unsolved problem on the public health level even though individuals can be treated and do recover. Why the various drugs come and go as the "in thing" is a complete mystery. Cocaine was once a highly popular intoxicant beginning in the 1880's and fading out in the 1930's, or even a little earlier. At one time we thought that it had been dropped because its dangers had been recognized and the temptation had been removed by the introduction of novocaine as a local anaesthetic. The recent return of cocaine shows how little we really know about the epidemiology of such substances, and the point is reinforced by minor epidemics of numerous other intoxicants.

Finally we come to a topic which is little dicussed but plays a large role in practical management of mental health services. I refer to the combined syndromes which never seem to fit easily into any one of the specialized services which now exist. Services for the mentally retarded are quite well-developed, in our area at least, and so, also, are those for the mentally ill. But where the two are combined in one individual the individual is likely to have difficulty being accepted in either type of service. The same holds true for convulsive disorder which is quite frequent in the retarded. The combination of drug dependence with psychiatric illness likewise poses a problem and there are various permutations of abuse of intoxicants, mental disorder, mental retardation, and convulsive disorder to be encountered in actual clinical practice. It has been my experience that many of these cases do well under treatment, and it is to be hoped that the future will see some special recognition for such combined syndromes. This does not exhaust the list of combined syndromes that make patients hard to place. Another example is that of psychosis combined with disabilities of age; nursing homes are ready to take the disabled but there is a problem when the case is complicated by psychosis.

Summary

As we look back on the events in psychiatry during the hundred years that have passed since the opening of South Oaks Hospital, we cannot help but be impressed by the spectacular advances which have taken place. What is more exciting is the fact that the pace of advance appears to be accelerating, at least at the technical and scientific levels. From my experience of just 50 years I can say that we have much to be grateful for. The statistics and fiscal data give some indication of what has happened, but one has to recall the actual cases themselves to feel the reality of what has happened. One has to recall the excitement deaths, the depressions for whom one could do almost nothing, the inabiltiy to control aggressive, noisy, denudative and incontinent behavior, the literal untreatability of schizophrenic patients who recovered or became chronic apparently by chance alone, the rampant tuberculosis and the endless flood of new cases that filled every ward. One has to recall all this and more to feel really how much improvement has taken place in the hospital treatment of mental illness. This leaves out all comment about the vast system of outpatient services which were essentially unknown even 50 years ago and which now care for the bulk of all pyschiatric cases.

As mentioned at the start of this paper, the improvements have not been uniform; some areas have advanced spectacularly and others have moved more slowly or not at all. The improved financing has accounted for the ability to expand the volume of services, the application of psychodynamics has provided a technique that is crucial to this work, and the development of new drug therapies has provided the tools for dealing with psychiatric disorder and its most distressing symptoms in ways that were undreamed of even a few decades ago. For the future we shall probably have to rely on technological advances if we are to see further improvements in these services; at least for the moment a major increase in financing does not seem to be a bright prospect.

The past has much to teach us and is perhaps our best lead as to what the future may hold. But in studying the past it is important to remember that we cannot apply current standards to what was done then. They were working under very different conditions and with an entirely different technology. Only the spirit and good will and dedication could remain constant through all that time and there are good indications that it really has done so. If we do better work it is because our tools today are better than those of the past tools which were developed by those who went before, and this holds true for the facilities in which we work and the resources which are available to us.

Selected Reading List

Amer. Psychiat. Assoc. Special Ed. Bd. *Amer. Psychiat. 1844–1944.* Columbia Univ. Press. N.Y. 1944.

Brill, Henry. The Future of the Mental Hospital and Its Patients. *Psychiatric Annals* 5:9 Sept. 1975. p 352–359.

Brill, Henry. Notes on the History of Social Psychiatry. *Contemporary Psychiatry* Vol. 21 No 6 Dec. 1980 p 492–499.

Brill, Henry. The Present and Future of the Psychiatric Hospital. In: *American Handbook of Psychiatry 2 Ed.* Vol. VII. Edited by Silvano Arieti and Keith H. Brodie. p 734–749 Basic Books N.Y. 1981.

Caplan, Ruth, B. *Psychiatry and the Community in 19th Century America.* Basic Books N.Y. 1969.

Deutsch, Albert. *The Mentally Ill in America.* Doubleday Doran Garden City N.Y. 1937.

Jones, Kathleen. *A History of the Mental Health Services.* Routledge and Keegan Paul, Boston, 1972.

Kraepelin, Emil. *One Hundred Years of Psychiatry.* Philosophical Lib. N.Y. 1962.

N.Y. State Department of Mental Hygiene. *Annual Reports* 1932–1960 Utica Press N.Y.

Pelner, Louis. Joseph Goldberger. *N.Y. State Jour. of Med.* Nov. 15, 1969 p 2936–2941 and Dec. 1 1969, p 3050–3055.

Schmidt, L.J. et al. The Mentally Ill in Nursing Homes. New Back Wards in the Community. *Arch. Gen. Psychiat.* 34:687–691 1977.

Spitzka, E.C. *Insanity.* Bermingham & Co N.Y. 1883.

Swazey, Judith P. *Chlorpromazine in Psychiatry.* M.I.T. Press Cambridge Mass. 1974.

U.S. Dept. of Commerce, Bureau of Census. *Patients in Hospitals for Mental Disease,* 1923. U.S. Gov. Printing Office, Wash. D.C. 1926.

Walters, J.H. Encephalitis Lethargica Revisited. *Jour. of Operational Psychiatry* Vol VIII. No. 1. p 37–46, 1977.

Ward, M.J. *The Snake Pit.* Signet P. 2496. New York 1946.

Chapter 2

ONE HUNDRED YEARS OF OCCUPATIONAL MENTAL HEALTH

Alan A. McLean, M.D.*

*Alan A. McLean, M.D., has served as Eastern Area Medical Director for IBM since 1973. He joined the company in 1957 as Chief Psychiatric Consultant, and was named Medical Director, Northeast, in 1971. A Clinical Associate Professor of Psychiatry at Cornell University Medical College, Dr. McLean is also an Associate Attending Physician at New York Hospital. Dr. McLean is a Fellow of the American Occupational Medical Association and was its President in 1978 and 1979. He is also a Fellow of the American Academy of Occupational Medicine and a member of the World Health Organization's Expert Advisory Panel on Occupational Health. He is a member of the New York County and State Medical Societies, the American Medical Association (where he was an Alternate in the House of Delegates), and the Permanent Commission and International Association on Occupational Health. He is a Fellow of the American Psychiatric Association and served for four years as Chair of its Committee on Confidentiality. He is a Diplomate of the American Board of Psychiatry and Neurology and is Board eligible in occupational medicine. In addition to 50 articles in professional journals and textbooks, Dr. McLean is author or co-author of eight books, the latest of which is *Work Stress* (Addison-Wesley). He also edits the Addison-Wesley Series on Occupational Stress. In 1975, Dr. McLean received the Health Achievement in Industry Award from the American Occupational Medical Association.

One cannot assess the history of occupational mental health activities without a brief review of the historical meaning of work to provide a frame of reference. For the work scene has been radically altered over the past century—altered many times. And its meaning to the individual has undergone many changes which in turn alter the ways in which mental health services can intervene on behalf of the worker.

After all, the changing nature and meaning of work have been the greatest force for the restructuring of American lives of any in our history.

Work

Let us go back in history. Most primitive societies knew no word for work. Many still do not today. That is, they make no distinction between work and non-work, between labor and leisure, between hunting and fishing and ritual dancing.

Indeed it wasn't until the Middle Ages that work as such developed a measure of differentiation and later of respectability. It eventually became honorable and even a "gateway to spirituality." Paul's stern admonition, "If any would not work, neither should he eat," was interpreted by Thomas Aquinas as meaning exactly that.

Protestantism fostered the development of capitalism "through its benevolent view of commercial activity in general and the money-making side of it in particular."[1]

Martin Luther leaned toward the opinion that worldly work was a necessity in the eyes of God. (Building on the base created by Luther, Calvin added a vital link: asceticism. With this key connection, work *and* money-making could be made fully legitimate—as long as you were careful not to enjoy either.)

These Calvinist-capitalist ideas of work were most

convenient for the leaders of the Industrial Revolution in England in the late 18th century. For the first time the worker became one facet in a mechanical complex. But there was no freedom of movement in a planned production process. As Adam Smith said, "The man whose life is spent in performing a few simple operations . . . has no occasion to exert his understanding or to exercise his invention in finding out expedients for removing difficulties which never occur . . . and generally becomes as stupid and ignorant as it is possible for a human creature to become."[2]

And soon after, came Frederic Turner's scientific management which said that there was "one best way" for performing every aspect of every job. This way could and was "scientifically" established and every worker must efficiently do his job by adhering to a rigid pre-established pattern.

This brings us well into the present century and to the time that the history of what we now think of as occupational mental health began. Taylor was espousing scientific management at about the same time Elmer Southard in 1920 was espousing industrial psychiatry. Southard had a brief but brilliant career as Director of the Boston Psychopathic Hospital and Professor of Neuropathology at Harvard. He encouraged the early work of Mary Jarrett, generally recognized as the founder of psychiatric social work, and of Herman Adler, both of whose early professional interests related to unemployment and personality and to "the mental hygiene of industry."

In 1919 Southard was asked by the Engineering Foundation of New York to study the possible psychiatric problems of workers who were discharged. They were interested in why engineers didn't make it in industry. In 1920 he reported that "60 percent of more than 4,000 cases reached discharge status through traits of social incompetence rather than occupational incompetence." In other words he was among the first to point out that it was not strictly job performance that led to people being fired.

In 1920 Southard wrote, "Industrial medicine exists, industrial psychiatry ought to exist. It is important for the modern psychiatrist not to hide his light under a bushel; he must step forth to new community duties . . . I think that we will have a place in the routine of industrial management, not as permanent staff, . . . but as consultants. The function of this occasional consultant would be preventive rather than curative of the general condition of unrest."[3]

And in the 1920's behavioral scientists from fields other than psychiatry commenced a series of contributions that continue to influence the psychiatrist who is a consultant in occupational settings. In 1923, Elton Mayo at the Harvard Physiology Laboratory was asked to investigate the high turnover in a textile mill. He observed that with the introduction of rest periods for workers, labor turnover decreased and employee morale rose. Then in 1924 Mayo began the widely heralded, decade-long study of working conditions at the Hawthorne plant of the Western Electric Company near Chicago. More than 20,000 employees were interviewed and a number of small experimental groups of workers were intensively observed as changes were made in their work situation. These studies showed the tremendous importance of individual interaction as a part of the work situation. They demonstrated that dissatisfactions arising in or out of the plant become entwined, influencing each other and affecting work productivity.

The Hawthorne studies concluded that a work organization has both economic and social functions. The output of a product may be considered a form of social behavior, and all the activity of a plant may be viewed as an interaction of structure, personality, and culture. If any of these variables is altered, Mayo noted, change must occur in each of the other two variables. Further, reactions to stress on the part of the individual employees arise when there is resistance to change, when there are faulty control and communication systems, and when the individual worker must make adjustments to his structure at work. Recent strong criticism of methodology hasn't changed the validity of these conclusions.

In 1922, 60 years ago, the first psychiatrist was employed full time in an American business organization. At the Metropolitan Life Insurance Company, Dr. Lydia Giberson had that pioneering distinction. Young at the time, Giberson stayed with Metropolitan until her retirement. She served in a variety of counseling roles to employees both in the medical department and later in the personnel department.

In 1924 a mental health service staffed by a psychiatrist, a social worker and a psychologist was introduced at Macy's department store. This approach was adopted from the early child guidance clinic model. In 1929, V. V. Anderson summarized the program in the first full-length book on industrial psychiatry. He and his team were concerned first with placement techniques and interviewing in the personnel office, but he became involved with employment tests; he studied workers' involvement in accidents and effected a remarkable reduction in the accident rate—particularly among delivery truck drivers. His program was terminated as a result of the Depression in the early 1930's. Temple Burling picked up the role at Macy's in the mid-30's. He was concerned with problems of morale and interpersonal relationships within various divisions of the company.

World War II drew on the skills of many psychiatrists to make innovative applications in the military and in our factories. As C. M. Campbell said, the war "swept the psychiatrist out of his hospital wards and his administrative routine."[4] His then contemporary observations were expressed in the hope that the psychiatrist would continue devoting more attention to that portion of social living which occupies the major portion of an employee's life—his job. And he concluded, "Industry turns out two main commodities, material goods and human satisfactions. The wholesome or unwholesome structure and the stability of our modern industrial community may well depend on the amount of attention given to the latter commodity."

Times change, the meaning of work changes, the economy changes. Psychiatry develops, the behavioral sciences expand, other mental health professionals gradually begin to develop more interest in occupational mental health.

(I do not wish to skip over the tremendous work during the First World War of the Industrial Fatigue Research Board in Great Britain or of the rehabilitation programs for those with "war neuroses" which followed, but time won't allow a really complete survey.)

The tremendous activity during the Second World War gave us a new understanding of men under the stress of war and the practical application of psychiatric insights to the problems of defense workers. The former set the stage for our current understanding of work stress. The latter involved consulting, diagnosis, and treatment in the work setting and produced conspicuous improvements in work performance.

Reviews in the *American Journal of Psychiatry* appeared annually from 1946 to 1966 on "psychiatry in industry."

As with the rest of psychiatry, the decade of the 1950's saw rapid expansion in areas of related interest and increased sophistication in practice.

Early in that decade the landmark study of the Glacier Metal Company by a team from the Tavistock Institute in London was reported. Here was a pioneering application of psychoanalytic concepts to the study of a work organization for more than three years by a team of some 15 researchers. That study was of the operation and dynamics of an entire factory and the changes in those operations which grew from the research. The subsequent work of both Jaques and the chief executive officer of Glacier proved a study model, parts of which were picked up by Harry Levinson and his team at the Menninger Foundation in their research at the Kansas Power and Light Company and by many behavioral scientists in their subsequent studies of work organizations from non-clinical frames of reference.

This was also the decade which saw massive expansion in "human relations" research from students in social psychology and industrial sociology. It saw the birth of the ongoing studies at the Institute for Social Research of the University of Michigan in industrial mental health from the theoretical framework of role theory which in turn influenced the work of many clinicians.

The Carnegie fellowships in industrial psychiatry continued at Cornell. At the Menninger Foundation seminars for industrial physicians and executives got underway as did seminars for Menninger residents. W. Donald Ross continued his teaching of industrial physicians at the University of Cincinnati and there began a burgeoning number of conferences, seminars and workshops on industrial mental health sponsored by international, national, state and local mental health associations.

Publications proliferated ranging from three textbooks (Ross 1956, Levinson 1957, McLean and Taylor 1958) to an explosion of articles in the popular press on related topics. The Group for the Advancement of Psychiatry prepared a definitive statement on the role of psychiatrists in industry.

Many national committees were active with those of the American Psychiatric Association, the American Medical Association and the Industrial Medical Association providing formal points of information exchange, the development of materials and official position statements.

Qualitatively, the 1950's saw the broadening of theoretical frameworks of psychiatrists and other clinicians who served as practitioners in and researchers of the world of work. Expanded psychoanalytic conceptualizations came from not only the Tavistock Clinic and the Menninger Foundation but from many individual practitioners in the growing body of postwar psychoanalysts. An increasing number of social psychiatrists also incorporated theory and method from the behavioral sciences in their work in industry—again at both a clinical and research level.

The 1950's, then, saw the conceptual seeds sown for most of today's activities in occupational mental health and with issues of work stress. This decade and the next were those in which today's practitioners were trained or in which their teachers were trained.

Contemporary Occupational Mental Health

Time does not allow detailed coverage of the decades of the 1960's and 1970's. Suffice it to say that activities on all fronts diversified, grew, in many areas, prospered. Nonmedical (and often non-clinical) people from many disciplines picked up various facets of what had been a fairly coherent field of occupational mental health. Psychiatrists, clinical psychologists, and occupational physicians all ran with the ball in many directions. Thus we now have employee assistance programs which avowedly offer support for employee mental health. Some are very good, for the most part staffed by psychiatric social workers. Many deal exclusively with the employee who is a problem drinker and these are for the most part staffed by alcoholism counselors with little or no clinical training. On the other hand, occupational physicians are becoming more sophisticated in dealing with psychiatric issues and many in human resources departments in employer organizations have gained a greater understanding of the psychodynamics of human behavior. A specialty field of organizational development in psychology has emerged. And the quality of work life movement is in full swing urging greater employee participation and decision making as it may relate to specific tasks and projects in which they are involved.

New popular banners fly which tend to place occupational psychiatry and occupational mental health in their shadow. Examples would be work stress and burnout. There are now thousands of stress management "experts" who seem to overshadow the more than 4,000 occupational physicians and the several hundred occupational psychiatrists with more traditional expertise and training.

The trends and issues in the past 11 years may be illustrated by the occupational mental health conferences held here at South Oaks Hospital and those of the Center for Occupational Mental Health at Cornell University.

At South Oaks, conferences on absenteeism, drug abuse in industry, the emotionally troubled employee, and work stress have been but four of 12 conferences in recent years. At Cornell, two conferences on the changing meaning of work, several on mental health and work organizations, one on occupational stress, and one on reducing occupational stress took place during the same years. The trend seems to be away from dealing with the mentally ill employee to various aspects of prevention and the current concern with stress issues.

This appears to parallel the changing interests in areas of concern to mental health professionals at large and to the broadening base of those who are delivering mental health services. For instance the Institute of Medicine of the National Academy of Sciences issued a report in November 1981, entitled, "Research on Stress and Human Health," following a very nearly two-year intensive study by more than 100 experts—its first report on such a topic.

Since it is not possible to fully develop additional historical material in this overview, I will conclude with an autobiographical account which covers one third of the past 100 years which are our concern today. It deals with half of the time span in which psychiatrists have worked in industry.

My own experience entering the field may not be unique, but it is illustrative. After specializing in aviation medicine and serving as an officer in charge of a flight surgeon's section in the Air Force, it became clear that psychiatric training would be necessary for me to truly understand any job like that. How else could I deal with the many psychosomatic reactions seen on sick call? How else could I understand and redirect the clearly misplaced feelings expressed so freely by commanding officers? And I was intrigued by the many cases of "flying phobia."

After completing a residency in psychiatry, I was fortunate to obtain a Carnegie Fellowship in industrial psychiatry at Cornell University. This offered one year in the School of Industrial and Labor Relations and another year of field experience under the supervision of social psychiatrists at Cornell University Medical College.

This educational experience, together with professional meetings and visits to work sites, convinced me that occupational psychiatry was to be my world. And so it has been for the past 30 years.

For sheer professional satisfaction, the diversified set of interests and experiences would be hard to beat: diagnostic consultations, brief psychotherapy, teaching, consulting with organizational management—the variety is constantly stimulating. Even today I have no way of predicting what the next phone call will bring: it may be a question about proposed company policy, or procedural change, or about an employee who is showing signs of disturbance.

And my involvement in the psychodynamics and psychopathology of working people has led to cooperation with professionals from many disciplines. The sophisticated occupational physician, the industrial sociologist, the social psychologist, the cultural anthropologist—all have skills applicable to the broad issues of the world of occupational psychiatry.

More Debt and Divorce Than Drugs and Delusions

In a 1978 *New York Times* feature article, Marilyn Machlowitz pointed out that psychiatrists who work for big organizations are more likely to encounter problems of everyday living than serious emotional disorders. A typical company psychiatrist, she said, will probably hear more about debt and divorce than drugs and delusions. To a large extent, she is correct.

Although individual counseling is a psychiatrist's most obvious function in the industrial world, it is not always the largest or the most significant part of the job. We also sometimes screen (but do not select) candidates for overseas transfer. We advise on company policies, conduct research on health-related issues, and educate management and supervisors about various aspects of human behavior.

The Organization as Patient

But, in fact, the psychiatrist's real patient is the organization itself. We must, therefore, apply classic methods of medicine to a human system of interpersonal relationships known as a work organization. We must be concerned with an initial set of observations; develop various tentative diagnoses; and formulate treatment hypotheses. Only then can we suggest therapy for the corporate personality.

Certainly, the "personality" of each work organization is unique. It is determined by products and services, as well as by its policies, practices, values, and style of leadership.

The corporate personality represents an important social influence for each employee. It also determines the course of action of the psychiatrist who is charged with influencing healthy behavior within the system. And, certainly, a legitimate role of the psychiatric consultant is to work toward influencing policies and practices that foster good health behavior and that contribute positively to the performance of an organization as a whole.

The Individual Employee as a Patient

Clinical contact with individual employees is a key part of the psychiatric consultant's job. This is an interesting slice of professional practice, because patients are usually seen much earlier in the course of their illness under this type of arrangement than they would be in a typical psychiatric setting. And since many of them are less seriously disturbed than patients seen in a mental health facility, therapy is often relatively brief. Prolonged treatment is not practical in an occupational health program, but a responsive patient-employee can make great strides in a short period of time, especially when his or her environment can be modified to reduce its stressfulness.

A psychiatric consultant may be called upon to help a patient returning to work after hospitalization for mental illness. Here, again, we must decide how to modify the work environment so that it is supportive of the employee's re-habilitation. Employers differ widely in their degree of willingness to be helpful in this regard, but many have the flexibility and motivation to sharply modify jobs and, at times, to create appropriate work for such an employee.

Occasionally, a psychiatric consultant will be called upon to help arrange for hospitalization of an employee, although this is usually a matter handled by community medical personnel. When a worker is away from a job because of psychiatric illness, the company's medical staff, especially the psychiatrist, may be asked to maintain contact with the patient's personal physician. The worker's therapeutic progress is monitored and, with his or her permission, may be explained to the employer.

Preventive Psychiatry

Moving beyond his or her fundamental clinical role, an occupational psychiatrist may have the opportunity to formally teach company managers. Such education is often aimed at early case findings and may include discussions of early signs and symptoms of emotional disturbance. These discussions, generally given in seminar form, are often directed toward increasing the group's understanding of various behavioral patterns.

Stress management workshops have become increasingly popular in executive circles. Such workshops allow participants to share and compare their perceptions of stressors and to discuss coping techniques at both an individual and an organizational level. They also provide the format for a discussion of stress reactions. The psychiatric consultant may lead or be otherwise involved with such activities.

Mental health education also includes informal periods of discussion with small groups of key executives. These sessions often help members of management understand the role that feelings play in their decision making.

Promotion, demotion, and job transfer are a way of life in the world of work. But such changes are often threatening and difficult for workers and their families to accept. The objectivity of the psychiatric consultant at such times has been clearly demonstrated and has proved useful to these individuals. For even without overt emotional disorder, supportive counseling at times of career change is often of great value to both the worker and the company.

Another role assumed by the psychiatrist in industry is that of a researcher: identifying characteristics within the work environment that adversely influence, or that support, healthy behavior. This type of investigation includes the gathering of epidemiologic data concerning the distribution of mental disorders in the employee population. It attempts to identify factors that produce unnecessarily high levels of anxiety. The organization psychiatrist also evaluates normally functioning employees to obtain a comprehensive picture of group motivation.

Additional Considerations

There is not time to discuss all the issues and activities that bear on occupational psychiatry. I have said nothing, for example, about disability determination. I have not discussed the current trends in Worker Compensation law that increasingly holds the employer liable for provoking a psychiatric disability. I have not talked about many of the broader issues of occupational safety and health today; nor have I addressed such important topics as confidentiality within the field.

References

1. Jenkins, D. *Job Power*, New York, Doubleday, 1973.
2. *Ibid.*
3. Southard, E.E. "The Modern Specialist in Unrest: A Place for the Psychiatrist in Industry," *Mental Hygiene*, 4:550, 1920.
4. Campbell, C.M. "The Psychiatrist and Industrial Organization," *American Journal of Psychiatry*, 100:286, 1943.

Selected Reading List

Campbell, C.M. "The Psychiatrist and Industrial Organizations," *American Journal of Psychiatry*, 100:286 1943.

Freedman, Alfred M., Kaplan, Harold I., Sadock, Benjamin J., editors, *Comprehensive Textbook of Psychiatry*. Chapter 47, "Occupational Psychiatry" by Alan A. McLean, M.D. Williams & Wilkins, Maryland, 1980.

Jenkins, D. *Job Power*, New York, Doubleday 1973.

Smith, Adam as quoted in Jenkins, above.

Southard, E.E. "The Modern Specialist in Unrest: A Place for the Psychiatrist in Industry," *Mental Hygiene*, Volume IV:550 1920.

Question-and-Answer Session

Audience:

Once you've been able to recognize bizarre or unusual behavior in an employee, what is the best route to take in order to convince this person to seek help?

Dr. McLean:

There are two legitimate times when one can directly approach such an individual. The first is when that person's work performance has been clearly affected. This is a legitimate concern, both of the employee and of the manager, and certainly is something to be addressed by that manager, whether or not there is a psychiatric problem. To talk about what you as a manager perceive to be a performance-related issue, and to explore with that individual the reasons why that performance may be deteriorating, and to raise the question if this be a medical problem would be appropriate. Talk in terms of referral to the company's medical department, not of referral to a psychiatrist, because that implies that the manager is making a diagnosis.

The second situation is when an employee asks for help; and people ask for help in lots of different ways. But beyond that, it becomes very difficult to intrude on an employee's privacy. Those are the two legitimate times one can suggest ways in which a person should get help.

Audience:

My experience has been that psychiatrists want to keep their patients working; they send them back to work with a note saying, "So-and-so is ready to return."

Dr. McLean:

You raise a question about the process of rehabilitation. Psychiatrists are anxious to have patients get back to work as early as possible, and I think we can all understand why. On the other hand, though, how many psychiatrists have spent much time in a factory or in a business operation? They know of the work situation generally from what their patients tell them, but they don't necessarily get an accurate report.

Each work organization has its own corporate personality. Some are willing to make all kinds of adjustments: modify the job, or modify the amount of time on the job.

All sorts of restrictions may be possible to help somebody get back to work during a rehabilitation period. Other employers, for many good and sound business reasons, are completely unable to do so unless that individual is close to fully well and able to fit into a productive slot. This varies widely from one employer to another.

Managers have a very difficult time when they get the note from the doctor saying that an employee is ready to come back to work and the manager recognizes that it is simply not possible. Sometimes one simply has to pick up the phone and call that doctor and explain the situation. This sometimes can be very helpful. The call should come ordinarily from the employer's medical department, and must, of course, take place with the employee's permission. But, in my experience, one can usually work out some form of accommodation. The company may have to say, "Sorry, the individual is totally unable to adapt to the job. Here's what I observe, and here's why." Talk to the employee about this quite candidly and be candid as well with the physician involved. An accommodation may be reached. At times, the individual will get well quite rapidly with the support of the work organization, his work group, and the task itself.

Audience:
Did I understand you to say that in this kind of a setting, the client is the organization?

Dr. McLean:
One of the many ways that a psychiatric consultant to an organization functions is to think of the milieu, the organization itself, as the client.

Audience:
Can you make some observations about the issue of confidentiality in that milieu?

Dr. McLean:

We are talking about two separate issues—both of them very germane to our discussion. First, when I speak of the organization as the client, I'm thinking of the role the psychiatrist has of influencing that organization by fostering policies and practices which allow the healthiest possible behavior and of providing the best possible benefits to allow people to get help early on.

The second area you raise has to do with confidentiality and is one which I think all physicians in occupational medicine, whether psychiatrists, occupational physicians, or internists, have to keep in mind. The code of ethics of the American Occupational Medical Association quite clearly speaks to this issue. Physicians do not discuss any aspect of an individual employee's medical problems without clear authorization from that employee. And even with permission, the physician does not discuss things like diagnoses with others in the organization. The physician speaks rather in terms of recommended work restrictions that stem from a medical problem. If someone has, for instance, a low back injury, the recommendation might be not to lift more than 20 pounds, or not to work in a position that requires bending and stooping.

The practical implication and application is appropriate and does not violate confidentiality. Confidentiality between the occupational physician, the employee, and the employee's private physician is absolutely paramount in any occupational health program.

Audience:

In industries that have Employee Assistance Programs, do you find that the employees use these services? What kind of feedback have you had from employees who have used them? Has it been positive or negative?

Dr. McLean:

The whole area of Employee Assistance Programs covers a tremendously wide range—from simple counseling and referral activities that may include referral to a lawyer, or a social agency in town, or a clinician or to a physician, to ongoing counseling for individuals with drinking problems and the like. Because they are so diverse it would be terribly difficult for me to try to generalize.

What I'm speaking from now are write-ups and experiences of people who are operating such programs. Some have been extraordinarily helpful to a large number of people. Some have gone overboard in terms of confidentiality, to the point of insisting on complete and total autonomy without any reporting to anyone in management or even in the occupational health department. EAP's range from good clinical programs to simple referral sources to fairly intricate programs that relate to specific disabilities, such as alcoholism. We're seeing a very rapid increase in the number of such activities, and I think it will be very interesting to see where the trend goes.

Audience:

We are in an era of declining private psychiatric insurance coverage. What are your views on the future of private insurance coverage by industry for psychiatric impairment?

Dr. McLean:

Given the skyrocketing costs of health care in the United States today, and given the increasing concern about the cost of these benefits by employers today, I think we are going to have a continuation of the recent trend of employers to look sternly at such costs. Given the national scene today, with a reduction in many benefits, we have some models already established that do not bode well for betterment of these benefits.

Those two trends I think may well put something of a cap on the pattern we've seen in the past years of increasingly generous benefits. My own view is that there are ways to control such benefit costs through peer review as well as other techniques. These benefits *can* have a bottom line cost-benefit experience that is very favorable.

Audience:

From your experience, how best can psychiatry demonstrate to industry that the psychiartric coverage that is on the decrease is a necessary part of medical coverage, and that it would be a wise move for industry to continue such coverage for its employees?

Dr. McLean:

I wish I had all the answers. There are many groups studying this particular problem. There are techniques, for instance, that can be very reassuring to insurance carriers and to employers, such as specific dollar amount maximum for each employee for outpatient psychiatric care. They could be generous, but at least there's a safeguard in terms of cost. Companies can control the type of professional help that is covered by such plans. They can control the number of visits to a practitioner with a review by an insurance carrier after a specific number. Some of these systems work very well, particularly when that review can assure that treatment is on target. Companies always have the opportunity to bring in a consultant to assess if the treatment is really necessary. Together with things like peer review there are ways that one can build in controls.

Audience:

Do you work through your medical department or are you separated from it? Do you have an office where an employee comes to you, or do you go to the employee in the field?

Dr. McLean:

For the most part, occupational health departments are located in the factory, in the plant or in the work location, and the employee comes in to that facility. About half of the people who come in to see me or my staff are looking for help. The other half are either applicants for a preplacement medical examination, those coming in for a routine periodic examination, or those referred in by management. Ordinarily employees looking for help come to us.

This raises a tangential issue which I alluded to briefly before, and that has to do with the knowledge of the workplace by the occupational physician. It's incumbent upon every physician to get out there and see what is going on on the shop floor and in the branch offices where the individuals are functioning and to identify factors in the work environment which may be physically or psychologically stressful; to have knowledge of what a specific task is when somebody comes in and says he's a "dispatcher," for instance. The physician must know specifically what that dispatcher does.

Physicians, whether they are in occupational medicine or in private practice, ought to know what the patient does in a lot more detail if they are going to provide advice that relates to that individual's employment.

Audience:

If there is indeed a lessening of insurance benefits or conservatism that's beginning to come about in industry, do you think that this will be followed by more intensive and elaborate in-house care?

Dr. McLean:

I don't know. There is a tremendous increase in the counseling activities of Employee Assistance Programs. Some have been sold to management based on exactly that premise: if counseling early on is available, there will be less need for more formal psychiatric care. I can't quite buy that premise, but some have been sold on that basis. Yes, occupational health programs are expanding, becoming more sophisticated, are beginning to get in to somewhat more therapeutic activity as opposed to purely preventive activity, but that's just beginning to take place. I think it's quite possible that there are going to be more definitive treatment services available by occupational health units as a result of this. It would be a logical assumption, and I could make a case for it.

Audience:
    What industries produce the highest amount of stress?

Dr. McLean:
    This question takes us back to that hackneyed old phrase, "What is one man's stimulus is another man's stress." Occupational stress—that is, a reaction to a stressor on the job—is so highly individual, we have to keep in mind an individual's vulnerability at the time of the stressor. What's going on in that individual's context, or environment, or psychological environment? What kinds of support systems does he or she have? What is the nature of the specific stressor for that individual? At least these three factors have to be considered, because we've seen many people in what most of us can think of as extraordinarily stressful situations who just float along like a cloud, getting by beautifully, with no symptomatic response, and we see another individual whose foreman looks at him cross-eyed and he becomes psychotic. It's that wide a continuum.
    Are there specific tasks that are thought to be more stressful than others? There was one interesting study in Tennessee that looked at occupations of people on first admission to psychiatric hospitals. They found secretaries and laborers as the two job categories who had the most "stress-

related disease," but that doesn't mean that all secretaries and all laborers are going to develop stress-related diseases.

It used to be thought that air traffic controllers had the most stressful jobs in the world. There was a very thorough study done at Boston University that found the only stress-related factor that separated air traffic controllers from a control group was a somewhat higher level of alcohol consumption, and a slight elevation, almost non-statistically significant, in blood pressure levels. This work laid to rest the belief that the air traffic controllers had very stressful work. They did identify many factors in the work environment, management techniques and so forth, that helped to make the job uncomfortable, but in terms of actual stress reactions, there were relatively few.

Audience:
Are specific studies being done that relate to the employment or re-employment of mature women?

Dr. McLean:
The American Journal of Psychiatry published a series of papers on women at work—studies of kinds of work, the number of people in various categories who are coming into the job market. We know that, depending on whose statistics you read, between 50 percent and 60 percent of women between the ages of 18 and 65 are in the work force today.

Audience:
But we know they're in the low-paying jobs.

Dr. McLean:
We're in a very difficult job market today. Look at the unemployment rates for various categories of people depending on the geography. Look at minority teenagers and you see a tremendous unemployment rate. In some parts

of Puerto Rico we're seeing a 50 percent unemployment rate.

If you're a bright young engineer coming out of college, you have no trouble at all. If you have no skills and are coming into the job market in the Detroit area, you're in trouble.

Audience:

Can employers institute changes that will help to alleviate the problem of unemployment?

Dr. McLean:

Some can and some are. Some are using things like flex-time or using two people to do one job on split shifts. We're seeing a lot of specialized training and re-training as technology changes, and we have rapid changes in technology today.

Audience:

Are there specific management techniques that you could say cause stress?

Dr. McLean:

I could tick off a whole host, and I'm sure everyone in this room could also. I would think of such things as not communicating with the employee about factors that relate directly to how that employee does his or her job. That is a very authoritarian and aristocratic management style. "Do it *this* way" can be very stressful for many people. We know that piecework is a lot more stressful than salaried work. Farther up the administrative ladder, there are a lot of things that a chief executive officer can do to provide a healthier, less stressful work environment; knowing and understanding the many alternatives he or she may have in implementing or recommending a policy is very important.

Chapter 3

ONE HUNDRED YEARS
OF PSYCHIATRIC NURSING

Helen M. Arnold, R.N., Ph.D., C.S.*

This year marks the 100th anniversary of South Oaks Hospital. Coincidentally, 1982 is also the centennial year of modern psychiatric nursing in this country.

Nursing of the mentally ill can, of course, trace its roots back to much earlier times—to the ancient Egyptians or to the Greeks who treated their emotionally depleted citizens

*Helen M. Arnold, R.N., Ph.D., C.S., is an Associate Professor of Nursing at Adelphi University and a clinical specialist in group and marital therapy at Mercy Hospital, New York. Dr. Arnold maintains a private practice in psychotherapy and is board certified in adult mental health therapy by the New York Nurses' Association. She holds a nursing diploma from the Ottawa Civic Hospital, Ontario; and Bachelor of Science degree and a Masters of Science degree from Adelphi University, and a Ph.D. from New York University. Currently, Dr. Arnold is a candidate for a postdoctoral certificate in psychotherapy and psychoanalysis at The Institute of Advanced Psychological Studies, Adelphi University. Dr. Arnold is the author of several articles on psychiatric nursing and is co-author of a textbook, *Mental Health Nursing: A Bio-psycho-cultural Approach* (C.V. Mosby Company).

and regulated that treatment in a way that the following quotation describes:

> As often as they had phrenetic patients or such as were un-hinged, they did make use of nothing so much for the cure and restoration of their health as symphony, sweet harmony and concert voices.[1]

Suggestion, kindness, occupational therapy, recreational therapy, music, hypnotism and something that was called "temple sleep" were all part of the milieu therapy of the day. Pythagoras traveled to Egypt where he observed the therapeutic measures in vogue there—specifically, cold baths, amusements and reading.[2] Even earlier, ancient Hindu writings contained in the Ayur-Veda (circa 1400 B.C.) classified mental illness, while another of the Vedas set down functions and qualifications for psychiatric nursing. The nurse was instructed to be "cool-headed, pleasant, kind-spoken, strong and attentive to the needs of the sick and indefatigable in following the physician's orders."[3]

In 1982, the American Nurses' Association's "Statement on Psychiatric-Mental Nursing" describes the functions of the psychiatric nurse as follows:

1. Responsibility for maintaining a therapeutic milieu.
2. Working with clients to help resolve some of their problems in living.
3. Acceptance of the surrogate parent role.
4. Supervision of the physical aspects of the clients' health needs, including responses to medications and treatments.
5. Health education, particularly in the area of emotional health.
6. Helping to improve the clients' recreational, occupational and social competence.

   7. Providing supervision and clinical assistance to other
      health workers, including other nurses.
   8. Psychotherapy.
   9. Involvement in social action related to the mental
      health of the community.

It has gotten somewhat more complex since 1400 B.C.

But, back to psychiatric nursing as it began in this
country. It had its real beginning in 1882 at McLean Hospital, a private psychiatric facility in Belmont, Mass., a
suburb of Boston. It was at McLean Hospital, known then
as McLean Asylum (by the way, the hospital is still very
active today), that the first training school for psychiatric
nurses was established.

Linda Richards, America's official "first trained nurse,"
graduated in 1873 from the New England Hospital for
Women and Children in Boston. She traveled to England
to meet Florence Nightingale who had already established
her famous St. Thomas Hospital School for Nursing in 1860,
after her service in the Crimean War. Before Florence
Nightingale's work, nursing of patients in hospitals was
done by family members, servants, religious orders or by
the other patients, or sometimes, even by the convicts from
local prisons.

Linda Richards was strongly influenced by Florence
Nightingale's work and returned to this country to organize
several mental hospitals and also to help establish the school
at McLean Asylum.

The real value of this school was quickly appreciated.
Within 10 years there were 19 American institutions providing training programs for psychiatric nursing. In 1886,
the hospital pioneered by making an affiliation with Massachusetts General Hospital whereby their nurses could
complete their senior year's training at McLean.

As early as 1906, nurse educators in this country began their pioneering work toward establishing affiliations in psychiatric nursing for *all* students enrolled in general hospital schools of nursing. However, it took quite a while to reach the goal of integrating psychiatric nursing theory and practice as part of the curriculum for all nursing programs in the United States—actually, the 1950's. And while in 1935, one half of the existing schools of nursing offered a course in psychiatric nursing, it was still pretty much the "stepchild" of nursing education until 1952 when psychiatric nursing became a required course for state licensure as a registered nurse.

It is *still* not the case in many other countries that psychiatric nursing is considered an integral or necessary part of the curriculum for nursing education.

To return to our history. Santos and Stainbrook,[4] in their article "A History of Nursing in the 19th Century," describe the roles and duties of the psychiatric nurse 100 years ago.

> Her duties included carrying out or assisting the physician with the psychiatric procedures of the day; administering such as whyskey, chloroform, and paraldehyde; and therapeutic measures such as hot and cold douches, showers, continuous baths and wet sheet packs. Various methods of inducing patients to take food also played an important part in the therapeutic measures practiced by physicians and nurses. However, the nineteenth century psychiatric nurse had very few psychological nursing skills at her command.[5]

"Habit training" was taught in psychiatric nursing courses in order to help nurses assist patients toward greater conformity or "acceptable behavior."[6] And Hildegarde Peplau notes that many of the common nursing activities seemed to reinforce an atmosphere of *mistrust* between already suspicious patients and their nurses. Such procedures included "sharp counts," "belt counts," periodic "bed checks," and periodic "body counts."[7]

From 1890 to 1930, this role for the psychiatric nurse did not change much; in fact, it probably didn't change substantially until after the 1950's, when the importance of the nurse-patient relationship was realized.[8] One psychiatric nursing text *was* published in 1920—Harriet Bailey's *Nursing Mental Disease*. But psychiatric nursing was largely a "custodial care" experience; the primary focus was on the patients' physical needs and on *control* of the patient. Such specialized psychiatric procedures as hydrotherapy, tube feedings and proper restraint procedures were added to the regular physical nursing measures. The "glimmerings" of some psychological intervention on the part of the nurse existed simply in the expectation that the nurse should maintain a good attitude of kindness, tolerance, and humaneness toward patients.

Nurses had few psychological techniques available to them and they were discouraged by the prevalent view that all mental illness was pretty much incurable. They were also stressed by the necessity of caring for large numbers of patients. Individualized care was virtually impossible and there was no evidence for the value of nurse-patient relationships.

As descriptive Kraepelian psychiatry gave way to psychodynamic concepts, the role of the psychiatric nurse also began to change. In private psychiatric facilities such as Chestnut Lodge in Maryland, nurses began to be acutely involved as participants in the treatment of mentally ill patients. And thus, they became more and more aware of the value of the newer concepts in psychiatric care and the need to integrate these concepts into the body of knowledge for education and clinical practice in nursing.

In the 1930's and 1940's, the somatic treatments of

mental illness became prevalent and nurses were quite involved in these. Such treatments as psychosurgery, deep sleep therapy, metrazol shock therapy and, as it was known then, electroshock therapy, all had their prominent eras. This upsurge in somatic therapies influenced the role of the nurse at the time. These therapies all required skilled nursing care, and Florence Nightingale had long since proved, through her hospital mortality statistics, the necessity of expert nursing services in carrying out any somatic therapy.

The psychiatric somatic therapies also added another element to the evolution of psychiatric nursing. As the early therapies did have some rate of success in improving the patients' condition, they became more amenable to psychological intervention and the demand for the mental health worker's interaction with the patient escalated.

The psychodynamic concepts useful in treating the mentally ill were gaining the ascendancy and the three that had the greatest influence on modern psychiatric nursing are psychoanalytic theory, interpersonal theory and, communications theory.[9]

World War II also influenced the development of modern psychiatric nursing. With a high rate of 43 percent of all Army discharges being attributed to psychiatric disability, the country became acutely aware of mental illness as a major public health problem. In 1946, the National Mental Health Act was passed. It authorized the development of the National Institute of Mental Health with its program for training psychiatric professional personnel, supporting psychiatric research, and providing aid to individual states for the development of mental health programs.[10] Since psychiatric nursing was one of the four professions specified in the training program, impetus was provided for the development of undergraduate and graduate programs in psychiatric nursing in many colleges throughout the country. A 1950 study by the National

League for Nursing coincided somewhat with the Mental Health Act and concluded that special training was required in psychiatric nursing.[11]

Graduate education of psychiatric nurses enabled nurses to begin to work on a colleague level with other members of the team who were also receiving advanced education through the intervention of the N.I.M.H. Social workers, psychologists, psychiatric residents and psychiatric nurses—the four professional groups singled out for training by the N.I.M.H.—often took classes together during this period. These graduate level programs in nursing also served to produce qualified teachers in psychiatric nursing for all sorts of programs—practical nursing, diploma schools, associate degree programs, baccalaureate, and graduate programs.

The new approach in psychiatric nursing began to emphasize the importance of the nurse's "therapeutic use of self" in the nurse-patient relationship and Hildegarde Peplau's seminal work *Interpersonal Relations in Nursing* was published in 1952. This helped to revolutionize the teaching and practice of psychiatric nursing and provided the theoretical framework for the development of the therapeutic role being practiced today.

Up to now, this has all been history out of books. What follows is from my personal experience.

I received my basic psychiatric nursing training in 1953 and I use the word "training" deliberately; it was more "training" than education. I was sent from my home school in Ottawa to a somewhat isolated, large psychiatric facility—a provincial hospital in Canada that was pretty much the equivalent of the state hospitals in this country.

The year 1953, at least in Canada, was immediately before the antipsychotic major tranquilizers came into common use. Those drugs changed the course of psychological treatment, milieu therapy, and community psychiatry.

But what was happening in Canada in 1953 was similar

to what happened in the United States. At that time, the halls still reeked of paraldehyde and I had scheduled experiences to learn to do such things as:

1. The nursing care of the lobotomized patient
2. How to supervise the admission of a patient—the cataloguing of all clothing and belongings—and since most patients came into the hospital to stay for a *long* time, there were numerous belongings to catalogue and keep track of
3. How to transport large groups of patients safely from one building to another
4. How to conduct the utensil count after meals
5. The proper procedure for continuous tub baths, wet sheet packs, showers, and other exotic forms of hydrotherapy
6. The intensive nursing care of the patient undergoing insulin coma therapy
7. Participating in OT and RT—supervising patients at dances and religious services
8. Tube feeding or IV feeding and complete bed care for the withdrawn, chronic schizophrenic patients who lay in the back ward dormitories; patients who had long since ankylosed into fetal positions
9. Preparation of the patient for "shock therapy"— since this procedure was quite different from the electroconvulsive or electrostimulative therapy procedure of today—it more often took the form of joining a "posse" that searched for the frightened patient who was hiding out to avoid his therapy
10. How to enter and leave a seclusion room safely— there wasn't just one "quiet room" on a unit. Each ward had several seclusion rooms and patients did not go in for a few hours of reduced stimuli, but spent months or even years in there.

It was a scene that wasn't too much different from and probably worse than that portrayed in the book, "One Flew Over the Cuckoo's Nest." I am afraid, if my own observations as a young student nurse are typical, that there was more than one "big nurse" present in each institution. But for the most part, there were dedicated, hardworking, overworked nurses trying to do their best with a situation that hadn't changed a great deal since the beginning of the century. Many of the old charts that I had to read as a student were of patients who had been in the hospital for 30 or 40 years and their admission diagnosis of "dementia praecox" was being changed to the more modern term "schizophrenia." Psychiatric nursing from the 1890's to the 1950's was, as Peplau has pointed out,[12] not a particularly attractive job. But in spite of it, the number of RN's working in psychiatric settings had grown from 471 in 1891 to 12,000 in 1951[13] and, of course, their number continues to grow.

Funds from the N.I.M.H. and the Bolton Act funds continued to support psychiatric nursing from 1946 until 1979, when the funds pretty much disappeared. There are still a few grants being awarded but the support is minimal now.

The 1960's and 1970's were something of a golden age for psychiatric nursing. Graduate education was expanding, and the integration of psychiatric nursing principles was being well established within the undergraduate curriculum. The community mental health movement was flourishing; psychiatric units were being opened in general hospitals. The liaison role for psychiatric nursing was evolving; clinical specialists became consultants to nurses in other areas of the hospital. Maternity, pediatrics and medical-surgical units all sought the expertise of the psychiatric nurse to help them deal with nursing care problems. Maxwell Jones's concept of the therapeutic community was influencing the nurse's role in milieu therapy. The prestigious psychiatric nursing journal, *Perspectives in Psychiatric Care,* began publishing in 1963; psychiatric nurses were publishing clinically focused articles in *Perspectives* and in several other journals. Many excellent textbooks in psychiatric nursing became available during this period.

The role of the psychiatric nurse was becoming more interesting and more challenging. Group dynamics, family therapy, and systems theory were concepts that were added, at first to the graduate curriculum and later, integrated on undergraduate level. Masters' degrees prepared nurses to become clinical specialists, proficient in the treatment modalities of group therapy, couples therapy and family therapy. Some nurses specialized in child psychiatry. The number of nurses with earned doctoral degrees was increasing and is still increasing. Approximately 2,000 nurses in this country now have doctorates.

The role of the clinical specialist in psychiatric nursing became clearly defined and standards and functions were described by the American Nurses' Association for both the professional nurse working in the psychiatric setting and for the master's level clinical specialist.

Another important development occurred in the mid-1970's to the late 1970's. A rigorous certification process became available for nurses to achieve certification either on a generalist level or as a clinical specialist. With different educational requirements, both levels have requirements that include written examinations, documented experience and supervised practice. The ANA publishes a directory of all certified nurses.

Also in the 70's, the American Nurses' Association's division on Psychiatric-Mental Health Nursing Practice established the "Council of Specialists in Psychiatric Mental Health Nursing." In 1979, there were 600 nurses listed as members. The Council has defined practice for clinical specialists as follows:

> Psychiatric and mental health nursing is a specialized area of
> nursing practice directed toward prevention, treatment and
> rehabilitative aspects of mental health care. Nursing treat-
> ments are based on assessment of need, diagnosis and eval-
> uation of progress. They include individual and group psy-
> chotherapy, family therapy, screening and evaluation, making
> house calls, conducting health teaching activities, providing
> support and medication surveillance and responding to clients'
> needs through community action, if appropriate.[14]

They also noted that the specialists work in a variety
of settings, such as acute and long-term care hospitals, outpatient clinics, community mental health care centers,
schools, offices, courts, and industry. A directory of all
members of the council has been published by the ANA.

The 1980's: What are some current issues in the
profession?

The widespread acceptance of the primary nursing
model in all areas of nursing presents particular problems
for psychiatric nursing. There is some conflict between the
principles of milieu therapy and those of primary nursing
which make it difficult to apply the model. Work needs to
be done to try to resolve some of these contradictions.

Nursing research is another area that must continue
to develop (the number of nurses with earned doctorates
is small but steadily increasing).

Another important issue has to do with direct third-
party payments for service. In December 1981, a third-party reimbursement plan was approved by one large health
insurance plan, the Defense Department's Civilian Health
and Medical Program of the Uniformed Services otherwise
known as CHAMPUS. After an experimental program providing for such reimbursement was authorized and carried
out in fiscal 1980, the Defense Appropriations Conference
Committee adopted a proposal to make the program permanent. It provided that state licensed nurse practitioners

and certified psychiatric nurses be considered regular CHAMPUS authorized providers. The sponsor of the amendment was Senator Daniel Inouye of Hawaii.[15] This is an encouraging start but much needs to be done in the profession to promote "the autonomy and validity of individual and private practitioners through political action, networking and advocacy for third-party reimbursement for nurses."[16]

What about the next 100 years for psychiatric nursing? With all due respect to the valiant and far-sighted nurses of the early days, we *did* get off to a very slow start in the first century of our history. Things really didn't get moving until about 30 years ago when education and clinical practice started to change rapidly. But the impetus for this change came mostly from the outside—from psychoanalytic theory, World War II, the Mental Health Act, psychotropic drugs and the Community Mental Health movement. They all influenced the development of the profession in profound ways.

I would like to speculate that the profession will continue to grow, to increase its body of theoretical knowledge, and improve its corpus or clinical experience. I would also like to suggest that psychiatrist nursing will finally have come of age and that, much more often, the stimulation for growth will come from the profession itself.

References

1. Manfreda, M.L. and S.D. Krampitz, *Psychiatric Nursing*, Ed. 10, Philadelphia: F.A. Davis Company, 1977, p. 33.
2. Ibid., p. 34.
3. Ibid., p. 33.

4. Santos, E. and E. Stainbrook, "A History of Psychiatric Nursing in the Nineteenth Century," *Journal of the History of Medicine and Allied Sciences*, Winter, pp. 40–74 (quoted in Kalkman, Marion and Davis, A.J. (eds.), *New Dimensions in Mental Health-Psychiatric Nursing*. New York: McGraw Hill Book Co., 1974, p. 6.

5. Ibid.

6. Peplau, H., "Reflections on Earlier Days in Psychiatric Nursing," paper presented at the Elizabeth Palmieri Memorial Lecture, Adelphi University, Oct. 12, 1981.

7. Ibid.

8. Lego, S. "Psychiatric Nursing: Theory and Practice of the One to One Relationship." A paper presented at a conference: "The State of the Art of Psychiatric Nursing" sponsored by the NIMH and held at Rutgers, the State University, New Brunswick, New Jersey, April 8–9, 1974.

9. Kalkman, p. 10.

10. Ibid., pp. 10–11.

11. Burgess, A. and A. Lazare. *Psychiatric Nursing in the Hospital and the Community*, Englewood Cliffs, N.J.: Prentice-Hall, Inc., 1973, p. 400.

12. Peplau, H. *Interpersonal Relations in Nursing*, G.P. Putnam Co., 1952.

13. Mereness, D. and C.M. Taylor, *Essentials of Psychiatric Nursing*, 10th edition, St. Louis, Mo.: C.V. Mosby Co., 1978, p. 57.

14. *Fact Sheet of the American Nurses' Association*, Division on Psychiatric and Mental Health Nursing Practice, Council of Specialists in Psychiatric-Mental Health Nursing.

15. *The American Nurse*, Vol. 14, No. 2, 1982.

16. Chaisson, M.G., candidate's statement, *The American Nurse*, Vol. 14, No. 3, 1982.

Chapter 4

MENTAL HEALTH AND THE FEDERAL GOVERNMENT—100 YEARS

Stanley F. Yolles, M.D.*

All civilized nations struggle to find ways to look after their mental casualties—the retarded, alcoholics, drug dependents, brain-damaged patients, and other emotional victims of society's stresses and strains.

In the United States the spirit of humanism has fluctuated from the high that attended the moral treatment era, roughly between 1830 and 1860, to the low that followed the indus-

*Dr. Stanley F. Yolles is a graduate of New York University Bellevue Medical Center where he received his M.D. degree in 1950. He was awarded the degree of Master of Public Health by Johns Hopkins University in 1957. Dr. Yolles served most of his professional career in the U.S. Public Health Services where he rose to the rank of Assistant Surgeon General (Rear Admiral) and was Director of the National Institute of Mental Health. In 1971, Dr. Yolles retired from the Public Health Service to become the Chairman of the Department of Psychiatry and Behavioral Science at the newly-organized State University of New York at Stony Brook, School of Medicine. In 1981, Dr. Yolles retired as Chairman and now devotes his activity to research and teaching. During the 1960's, he was intimately associated with developments in the field of mental health and was an active proponent and implementor of new developments in the field of psychiatry and behavioral sciences.

trialization of the economy after 1860. After World War II a painful and gradual return to humanism occurred. The evolution of Social Security legislation and the abandonment of social Darwinism and the philosophy that individual initiative alone can solve all hardships represented the major social and ideological shifts of the period. The level of care and treatment of the mentally ill has paralleled each change.[1]

The middle of the 19th century saw a wave of reform initiated by Dorothea Dix's attempts to improve services and hospitals for the mentally ill. Miss Dix mounted her white charger in 1841. Her campaign was successful in establishing 32 additional state hospitals and led directly to the involvement of the Federal government in mental health service delivery.

As a result of Miss Dix's successful campaign, St. Elizabeths, the first Federal mental hospital, was established in the District of Columbia in 1855.

The dedicated, devoted, and determined Dorothea's greatest achivement, however, was to convince Congress in 1854 to set aside more than 10 million acres of Federal land for land grants to be used by the states to provide funds for the indigent mentally ill. Although the bill was vetoed by President Franklin Pierce, who felt that care of the handicapped was none of the business of the Federal government, the work accomplished by Miss Dix became a part of the American conscience and tradition.

Federal interest and its overt expression in funds for capital expenditures dwindled, and by 1968, when taken over by the National Institute of Mental Health, St. Elizabeths had deteriorated into an antiquated, dirty and dilapidated institution.

Waves of immigration in the latter half of the 19th century and beginning of the 20th century led to further Federal involvement in mental health services. Today we applaud Emma Lazarus' words on the Statue of Liberty; however, immigrants were not always welcomed to our shores.

Studies carried out in the first 20 years of the 20th century showed a higher percentage of foreign born than native born among those admitted (as first admissions) to New York State hospitals. The mental health implications associated with foreign immigration helped bring about a greater awareness that mental diseases and defects constituted a national health problem. From 1900 to 1921, the foreign born constituted 15 percent of the general population but comprised 46.6 percent of all first admissions to New York State mental hospitals.

In 1904, Dr. Thomas W. Salmon, of the United States Public Health Service, was assigned with others to the USPHS hospital on Ellis Island to assist in the mental examination of immigrants. The group worked at developing techniques for identifying the mentally handicapped under the difficult conditions posed by the need to examine several thousand persons in one day.

This was at best difficult, and at the worst, impossible, because of the short time available for the examination and the fact that the immigrants spoke a multiplicity of languages. The detection of insanity, chronic alcoholism, epilepsy, and other diseases naturally depended a great deal on the history. This was not readily available.

The detection of mental retardation imposed a different problem. Each examiner had to become adept at asking a few questions in numerous languages. At first there was no technique available to detect retardation except in its grossest forms.

The introduction of the Binet test in 1908 renewed interest in the diagnosis of mental retardation by means of tests. It soon became apparent to the Public Health Service,

however, that the Binet system with its standards for diagnosis was not applicable to immigrants. It was a long time
(in some cases not until very recently) before this was appreciated by some workers outside of the Public Health
Service which had concluded that about 85 percent of certain
groups of immigrants were retarded.

The Service soon came to the conclusion that persons
with equal native ability coming from different cultural
strata and with different educational and environmental
backgrounds varied greatly in their ability to perform in-
telligence tests. It was, therefore, necessary to interpret
each group with these concepts in mind.

"The passage of the Prohibition Amendment indirectly
involved the Federal government in another need for mental
health services. In 1916 there were five Federal prisons
housing some 5,000 prisoners. By 1929 there were 12,000
prisoners in the same five prisons built to house 7,000 inmates. Four thousand or more of the inmates were violators
of the liquor laws."[2]

On the assumption that there is a considerable element
of mental abnormality concerned in one way or another with
conduct disorders, delinquency, and crime, the U.S. Public
Health Service accepted the challenge and undertook to address the problems of narcotics addiction, crime, and delinquency in prisons.

The principles that were developed for the treatment
of Federal prisoners stressed the provision of medical, surgical, and psychiatric measures for the correction of re-
mediable disabilities.

From 1930 to 1940, overcrowding in the prisons was
reduced, and medical housing, equipment, and staffing were
modernized. Regular and reserve officers of the U.S. Public
Health Service were chosen for their psychiatric ability and
interest in penology, and were assigned to the several
institutions.

A more important impetus to a federal mental health program, however, came from another direction—and something of an unexpected direction at that. Following passage of the Harrison Narcotics Act in 1914, the cause or causes of narcotic addiction and its treatment and cure became a matter of serious concern to the medical profession and government alike. The number of addicts in the United States was not accurately known, but it was commonly thought that they were relatively numerous.[3]

The more that narcotic drug addiction was studied, the more it became apparent that there were psychological and social as well as biological implications.

Addiction was recognized by many as a neglected medical problem of such importance that it could be dealt with adequately only at the Federal level. In 1928, a bill was introduced in Congress to authorize construction of two hospitals for the confinement and treatment of persons addicted to the use of habit-forming drugs. The bill was signed into law in 1929.[4]

Lexington, Kentucky, was chosen as the site of the first hospital and Fort Worth, Texas, as the second. Lexington was originally known as the first U.S. Narcotic Farm, and was opened in 1935. Fort Worth opened in 1938. Dr. Lawrence Kolb, a psychiatrist and a distinguished authority in the field of narcotic addiction, was the first medical officer in charge at Lexington. This hospital contained a research unit so that investigations of addiction could be carried out. The hospital names were later changed to eliminate the words "narcotic farm," becoming known as U.S. Public Health Service Hospitals.

The act also created a Narcotics Division in the Public Health Service to administer the hospitals and to carry out research on addiction and rehabilitation of addicts. Very soon it became apparent that although addiction itself is a physiological phenomenon, its etiological roots extend deeply into the personality of the victim. In studying these conditions and in advising the states with regard to programs for the control of addiction, it was inevitable that to a greater and greater extent the consultation centered about problems of mental health and mental disease. The new Narcotics Division lasted only a year as a formal entity, and in 1930 its scope was enlarged to include studies related to the causes, prevalence, and means for the prevention and treatment of mental and emotional disorders. The Federal government was fully in the mental health field for the first time, and the name of the Narcotics Division was changed to the Division of Mental Hygiene.

During the 1930's, mental health activities were consolidated and an organized Federal program begun. The U.S. Public Health Service thus was involved with states and communities not only in cooperating to provide treatment and facilities for addicts, but it was involved also in studies of the cause, treatment, and prevention of mental illness.

Four years after passage of the Harrison Narcotics Act, we were drawn into World War I. General John J. Pershing, Commander of the American Expeditionary Forces in that "war to end all wars," sent the following cablegram to the U.S. Army Chief of Staff on July 18, 1918: "Prevalence of mental disorders in replacement troops recently received suggests urgent importance of intensive effort in eliminating unfit . . . prior to departure from U.S. . . . ."

"Black Jack" Pershing placed the responsibility for resolution of the problem where it belonged: back home with the professionals. There were three leaders: Dr. Thomas Salmon, first medical director of the citizen's National Committee for Mental Hygiene and an early president of the American Psychiatric Association; Dr. Taliaferro Clark; and Dr. Walter Treadway. These three physicians, following their experiences with military psychiatry in World War

I, developed the recommendation which resulted—*eventually*—in the establishment of the Division of Mental Hygiene in the United States Public Health Service.

Clark and Treadway proposed a program for the government based on their experiences in World War I. That military plan included early recognition of mental and emotional disturbances; prompt treatment; continuing treatment by psychiatrists at base hospitals; hospitals at embarkation and debarkation ports; military hospitals in the United States serving as training schools; psychiatrists attached to all military divisions to advise medical and line officers; and elimination of the mentally retarded from the armed services.

However, although this system was operative and successful in the military setting, it was forgotten as soon as the troops came home. The proposal to establish a Mental Hygiene Division in the Public Health Service—first put forward in 1914—was not approved until 16 years later in 1930.

The written—but unpublished—plan set forth by Clark and Treadway in 1919 (known to those who saw it as Volume X) did not surface again until World War II when the British utilized it as the basis of psychiatric procedure. Not until the end of World War II, with the passage of the Mental Health Act of 1946, did the Federal government accept responsibility commensurate with the 1919 proposal.

Simultaneously, in the years between the two World Wars, the idea of psychiatry for any community outside the military was an idea whose time had not yet come.

As a step in preparing for possible involvement in another war, the Congress adopted the Selective Service Act of 1940; the military took another look at Volume X and men eligible for the draft received psychiatric screening as a routine part of their medical examination.

Albert Glass (1970) traces the history of military psychiatry to contend that "the origins and development of the community mental health movement have been strongly influenced by the practical insights of military psychiatry." One well-accepted principle of community psychiatry—the frequency of psychiatric disorder is related to social and environmental circumstances—is a perfect example of lessons learned painstakingly through military experience in one war and relearned in later wars.

The principles outlined by Salmon (1919) in World War I—proximity, immediacy, and expectancy—were largely forgotten, only to be rediscovered late in World War II. The Korean War resulted in recognition of the additional principle of community—individual problems were often manifestations of problems within the community. These principles were applied early during the Vietnam War.

In 1936, Dr. Treadway was succeeded as Chief of the Division of Mental Hygiene by Dr. Lawrence Kolb, a psychiatrist who had contributed so much to the understanding of narcotic addiction. It was during Dr. Kolb's administration that the idea of a National Neuropsychiatric Institute came into being. He envisioned the Institute as having both clinical and basic research facilities for the comprehensive study of mental and nervous diseases. He further advocated that the Institute should be able to allocate funds to competent research groups throughout the country after appropriate review. Kolb redrafted his proposal in the form of a bill to be introduced in Congress, but just as it looked as though there might be favorable results, World War II intervened and the bill was never introduced.

It was dismaying to both professionals and lay leaders to learn how many of our young men had emotional disabilities which disqualified them for service. Between January 1942 and June 1945, according to Dr. Bill Menninger, out of approximately 15 million examinations for inductions into the Armed Services in World War II, almost two million individuals were rejected for neuropsychiatric disability. To put it another way, for every 100 men examined, 12 were rejected for neuropsychiatric reasons. For every 100 rejections for all causes, neuropsychiatric rejections accounted for 40 percent.

The manpower loss, in the army alone, before and after induction, totaled more men than were assigned to the Pacific Theatre of Operations during the entire war.

As Robert Felix put it in 1967, "If these young men were representative of the nation as a whole, what would be the absolute figures for the mental and nervous impairments of the entire population? At least one study projected the figure of one American in 10 who needed psychiatric help of some kind."[5]

In 1945 it appeared that the time was ripe for strong public action in the field of mental health. The data on mental illness and disability were well-documented and known by many informed people both in and out of Congress. There was serious concern about the implications for the future if positive action was not taken. In 1945, Representative J. Percy Priest of Tennessee, in the House of Representatives, and Senators Claude Pepper of Florida, Lister Hill of Alabama, Robert A. Taft of Ohio, George Aiken of Vermont, Robert La Follette, Jr., of Wisconsin, and a number of others from both sides of the aisle in the Senate introduced identical bills in the two Houses, the stated purpose of which was "to improve the mental health of the people of the United States . . . "

These bills set forth three general purposes: to support research on the cause, diagnosis, and treatment of neuropsychiatric disorders; to provide for training of personnel through the award of fellowships to individuals and grants to institutions; and to provide financial aid to the states to establish clinics and treatment centers, as well as the provision of pilot and demonstration programs in the prevention, diagnosis, and treatment of mental and emotional disorders.

An interesting sidelight on the rapid-moving events of this time should be noted. The President signed the bill on July 3, 1946, and Congress adjourned the next day, July 4. This resulted in a law on the books authorizing a vigorous program in mental health research, training, and service; but no funds were provided to implement the Act. It was thought essential that there be an early meeting of the National Advisory Mental Health Council (which was promptly appointed as the law provided), but there were no funds to call a meeting of the body, once created. Those responsible for getting the program underway then did what program directors and scientific investigators have done before and since; the rounds of the private foundations were made (by Dr. Felix) in an effort to obtain sufficient assistance at least to call a meeting of the Advisory Council. In New York City, the Greentree Foundation (no longer in existence) listened sympathetically to the needs for funds and awarded a grant of $15,000 for this purpose. It has always seemed particularly significant that the National Institute of Mental Health which awarded funds to so many grantees for training and research purposes had its origin in a grant made by private philanthropy

Even though the National Mental Health Act of 1946 was easily enacted into law, the Act was something of a step out-of-step. Congress had prescribed for the symptoms before having the diagnosis.

As a result, the Mental Health Study Act of 1955, signed into law by President Eisenhower on July 28, 1955, some nine years later, authorized an appropriation to set up a Joint Commission to survey the resources and make recommendations regarding the status of mental health and mental illness in the United States. This had never before been attempted on a national basis.

World War II had marked a turning point in American psychiatry. After the war, public interest was focused on the "snake pits" of the public mental hospitals which the war had created through depletion of scarce personnel. The State Mental Hospital system had become so rigid that the task of the Joint Commission (even in trying to find out what was actually happening in these hospitals) was as difficult as trying to carve Mount Rushmore with an ice pick.

Six years and 10 books later, the Joint Commission on Mental Illness and Health delivered its report in 1961. The report recommended increasing support for mental hospitals; making available emergency psychiatric care; providing intensive treatment of acutely ill mental patients in clinics, general and mental hospitals; expanding the number of outpatient clinics; and establishing general hospital psychiatric units. The report urged that smaller state hospitals (with 1,000 beds or less) be converted into intensive treatment centers, and that state hospitals with more than 1,000 beds become centers for long-term care of physically and mentally ill people. The report stressed aftercare and rehabilitation services and encouraged day and night hospitals. The Commission proposed that the cost of the program be shared by Federal, state and local governments.

As a result of the report, a committee was established by the President to make recommendations on implementation. The committee had representation from N.I.M.H., the Veterans Administration, the Council of Economic Advisors, and the Bureau of the Budget.

The President accepted the new recommendations of his committee. On February 7, 1963, for the first time in the nation's history, a President of the United States—John F. Kennedy—sent a message on mental illness to the Congress, because, as he said, "the problem is of such critical size and tragic impact and the susceptibility to public action is deserving of a wholly new national approach." He proposed legislation for a "bold new approach" through establishment of community mental health centers, while helping state mental hospitals to improve their treatment programs through improvement grants of up to $100,000 a year for 10 years and grants for in-service training to upgrade the staffs.

If one looks further into the data on which President Kennedy based his message to Congress, the record becomes far worse than dismal. It was a dreadful situation. Only 28 percent of the state mental hospitals in 1961 had been able to meet the criteria for accreditation by the Joint Commission on Accreditation. Even worse, the rate of accreditation was declining. The proportion of all public mental hospitals rated as "nonacceptable" had risen from 14 percent in 1950 to 28 percent in 1961. Also in 1961, more than one-third of the mental hospitals in the United States were more than 75 years old and many of the original buildings were still in use.

In 1963, the most powerful advocate of a national community mental health system was President Kennedy.

Before the end of the year 1963, the Congress had responded with passage of the Community Mental Health Centers Act. The National Institute of Mental Health was assigned the authority to administer the Act, establish guidelines for states and communities and—most importantly—draft regulations to be met by applicants for Federal funding support of proposed community mental health centers.

I think it pertinent in 1982 to quote the 1963 definition: "A comprehensive community mental health center is a multi-service community facility designed to provide preventive services, early diagnosis and treatment of mental disorders, both on an inpatient and outpatient basis, *and to serve as a locus for aftercare of discharged hospital patients.*"

As adopted, the Community Mental Health Centers Act provided for funds to support construction of community mental health centers. Period. The original proposal had also included appropriation of funds to help finance the initial cost of staffing the centers, but responding to objections from the A.M.A., that was eliminated. Two years later, the educational process had progressed to the point that Congress amended the legislation to include staffing funds.

Bit by bit and piece by piece—since 1963 the act has been amended seven times—other requirements were added to extend the mental health services program into a number of areas including children's services, alcoholism, and drug abuse.

But at no time was any strong voice raised from inside government or from professionals or others outside to plead the case for the chronic patient.

The intent of the Congress was that this was to be a continuing program, rather than a pilot demonstration; although the Congress (which rarely, if ever, signs a blank check) continued to set time limits for funding and continued to request states and communities to assume the basic funding responsibility.

By 1970, it was clear to officials of the National Institute of Mental Health that the White House intent concerning the community mental health centers program differed from that of the Congress. To be blunt about it, the Nixon administration wanted to kill the program.

As you know, Congress has the power to appropriate funds, but the funds are allocated by the Executive. In 1973–74, the President chose not to allocate community mental health center funds for the next fiscal year. Funds already committed would be released, but there would be no new funding. But that ploy did not succeed. Over the years, in order to improve their programs and communicate with one another, the directors of the community mental health centers had formed a national organization; and this organization went to court. The center directors won their suit and the funds were belatedly restored to the program.

This victory provided a stimulus to the entire mental health community and stimulants have side effects. One of the major effects was to revitalize Congressional interest in what the Congress again stated was a continuing program.

A number of other agencies of the Department of Health, Education and Welfare also support or influence mental health programs. The Food and Drug Administration regulates the development and use of all drugs, including drugs used in psychiatry. Some NIH research institutes, notably the National Institute of Neurological Diseases and Stroke, and the National Institute of Child Health and Human Development, support mental-health related research. In the service area, the Social Security Administration reimburses citizens who qualify under Medicare and Medicaid for some mental health expenses. The Department of Education, prior to its proposed demise, funded projects related to mental health. The Office of Child Development, in the Office of the Secretary, funds service demonstration projects which may include mental health services.

Outside D.H.E.W., mental health activities exist throughout the executive branch. The Department of Defense supports psychiatric care for active duty personnel. Psychiatric research is carried out at the Army Medical Center, Walter Reed Hospital in Washington, D.C., and at the Naval Medical Center in Bethesda, Maryland. The Veteran's Administration has a budget of billions for its network of hospitals and clinics for ex-servicemen; approximately 20 percent of this total is earmarked for V.A. psychiatric hospitals. In addition, the V.A. supports psychiatric training and research in its facilities. The Justice Department investigates and controls the production, distribution, and use of dangerous drugs, including several drugs used in clinical psychiatry through its Drug Enforcement Agency. Criminal justice grants from the Justice Department's Law Enforcement Assistance Administration (L.E.A.A.) often have mental health significance.

Support for mental health related services and research also originates in the alcohol-prevention program of the Department of Transportation, and other executive branch agencies.

Deinstitutionalization is a term which came into use in the 1970's, and means different things to different people. To the average mental health professional it means the release of mental patients back to community living as soon as the patient's condition will allow. To the community resident and taxpayer it means having his neighborhood overrun by strange, peculiar acting, and possibly dangerous people. To the state legislator it means smaller budgets for the mental institutions and more complaints from his constituents if their community is involved. To the patient it means release from the hospital and early return to living in the community.

According to Gerald Klerman in 1977:

> The policy of deinstitutionalization fostered an interesting alliance of three groups. One group included progressive leaders in the mental health field who extrapolated from research demonstrating the value of outpatient treatment for acute episodes, and reasoned that what was good for acute schizophrenics would be good for chronic schizophrenics. The second group included civil libertarians, who were genuinely concerned with the abuses of "total institution." The third group included the fiscal conservatives in states such as California, who felt that there was budgetary gain in transferring hospitalized patients into community settings where they would be under the aegis of public welfare agencies, rather than the responsibility of the Department of Mental Health. [6]

This major public policy decision was made almost simultaneously in about 40 states in the late 60's.

In the absence of an adequate network or adequate funding for the development of aftercare facilities, community residences, halfway houses, sheltered workshops, and day treatment centers, large numbers of patients are relegated to "lives of quiet desperation" in welfare hotels and in segregated neighborhoods. They are subsisting on minimal incomes from social welfare or disability payments, and receiving poorly-monitored, often poorly-prescribed psychotropic medication.

As the U.S. Comptroller General's report on deinstitutionalization put it:

> A basic problem at the Federal, state, and local levels is that those agencies primarily responsible for the mentally disabled do not have the funds needed to develop adequate, comprehensive, community-based care systems for the mentally disabled. In addition, they do not have all the responsibility for regulating or monitoring the standards of care in communities. Therefore, they have approached deinstitutionalization by relying on the many social, welfare, and other programs that affect such target groups as the poor, the aged, children, or the disabled, to accomplish deinstitutionalization individually without any central guidance or management. [7]

As a result of the criticism levelled by the General Accounting Office, the National Institute of Mental Health developed an extensive human services planning program focusing on the needs of former hospital patients. This new Community Support Program envisaged intensified interagency planning at the Federal level and fiscal partnerships of Federal, state and local agencies to support direct services to the target. On February 17, 1977, President Carter signed Executive Order number 11973 establishing the

President's Commission on Mental Health. In remarks at the formal signing ceremony, the President, and his wife, displayed a sensitivity to the needs of the mentally ill, expressing a desire to provide adequate care for those who need it.

Broad in scope, this charge called for an assessment of the mental health system, not just as it existed, but projected over the next 25 years, with particular emphasis on the role of the Federal government in providing treatment for the underserved. Despite the conviction of mental health professionals that increased expenditures were needed, there were no allusions in the Executive Order to additional funding. Indeed, remarks made at the signing ceremony gave the impression that coordination, redistribution, and more efficient usage of existing resources could provide an adequate solution.

The President's Commission Report was submitted in April 1978, and it was soon on its way to influencing prospective legislation. Immediately after its appearance, the Secretary of what was then Health, Education and Welfare (now Health and Human Services, humorously called H-2-S), established an Interagency Task Force to analyze the implications of the report's recommendations, and to propose legislation that would be responsive to the Commission's recommendations and intent.

The future of community mental health in part, depended on the fate of the Mental Health Systems Act (PL 96-398), passed by Congress on October 7, 1980, based on the findings of the H.E.W. Task Force. It is difficult to predict the influence of the Act. The Mental Health Systems Act seemed to have something for everyone. It gave state mental health authorities more power and a little more money. It centralized control of planning for service delivery in the health system, not an unmitigated blessing from some mental health viewpoints. The legislation endorsed the community mental health concept, and made it easier to start new community mental health centers. To meet criticisms of deinstitutionalization, the legislation authorized expenditures on services in the community for the chronically mentally ill. In addition, it provided funds for new services targeted to the previously underserved priority populations. The interests of a variety of constituencies—minorities, Indians, women, advocates of prevention, community mental health center workers, displaced employees within institutions—were recognized in one way or another.

Since then, a new administration has taken office, and a new Congress, highly conservative fiscally, is in place. In the past, mental health legislation had its friends in Congress, and in fact President Ford's veto of mental health appropriations in 1975 was actually overridden by the Congress. Now the Senate is controlled by the Republican party, and it is unlikely that a Reagan veto would be seriously challenged.

You are all aware of the 1981–1982 and 1982–1983 budgets submitted by the Reagan administration. Behavioral science research has been drastically curtailed and all mental health service training has been eliminated. The Mental Health Systems Act has disappeared into oblivion. The administration acted, in the words of Senator Daniel P. Moynihan, to wipe out 30 years of social legislation with the stroke of a pen. Even though we are still a long way from an equitable, humane, and effective system for community care of the chronic mental patient, mental health programming has been turned back to the states by means of block grants at reduced levels with few Federal strings attached. Future mental health programs were in the planning stages—how and when and if they appear and how they are implemented—is only partly a responsibility and function of mental health professionals. Society at large in the United States, through its legislation and its government, will decide the issue.

Our review of the history of Federal involvement in mental health has taken us along a winding path. Events of national significance—war, immigration, narcotics control, prohibition—had correlates in human problems. As the human problems came to political awareness, solutions emerged. Often the solutions were piecemeal, and directed toward the treatment of individuals in distress, but eventually a clear national program began to evolve.

As any student of history knows, progress and regression within the practice of mental health have always been related to the expressed attitudes of the general population. In times of collective humanism, mental health programs have advanced; in times of political doubt, suspicion, and reaction, they have come under attack and regression. In the field of mental health, especially, events of the past 15 years illustrate how closely the provision for and delivery of mental health services is related to the national political climate.

The "bold new approach" signaled by one President may be side-tracked or even demolished by another, but the plain facts of everyday living will continue to reinforce public and professional demand for humane and sensitive mental health programs in the United States.

References

1. Greenblatt, Milton. *Hospital and Community Psychiatry*, November 1979, Vol. 30 (11), pp 760–762.
2. Williams, Ralph C. *The United States Public Health Service, 1798–1950*, Commissioned Officers Association of USPHS, 1951.

3. Felix, Robert H. *Mental Illness Prospects and Projections*, New York Columbia University Press, 1967.
4. Ibid.
5. Ibid.
6. Klerman, Gerald L. *Federation Proceedings*, Vol. 36 (10), p 2352, 1977.
7. *Report of Comptroller General of the U.S.*, 1977. U.S. Government Printing Office.

Chapter 5

PRIVATE PSYCHIATRIC HOSPITALS— THE LAST 100 YEARS

Leonard W. Krinsky, Ph.D.*

A comprehensive report on private psychiatric hospitals must first take into account that the myth about the private hospital is a more realistic concept for the general public than is the reality of what private psychiatric hospitals have been and are.

*Leonard W. Krinsky, Ph.D., is a graduate of Temple University, and the University of Arkansas, and was awarded his doctorate in Clinical Psychology from Adelphi University. He has been involved in psychiatric hospital work for much of his professional career with a period of time when he was employed as a school psychologist in Suffolk County. In addition he has been in private practice for many years. Over the years he has worked closely with the Nassau and Suffolk County Police Departments and has been appointed Police Surgeon by both. In addition he has a special interest in the evaluation of candidates for religious vocations. He is a consultant to the Diocese of Rockville Centre.

Dr. Krinsky is a Diplomate in Clinical Psychology, is Administrator and Director of Psychological Services at South Oaks Hospital and Secretary of South Oaks Foundation. He is also Associate Professor of Clinical Psychiatry in the School of Medicine at the State University of New York at Stony Brook, and Associate Professor of Clinical Psychology at the Institute for Advanced Psychological Studies at Adelphi University.

Consequently, let me first discuss the myth which, in any event, is probably more interesting than the reality. The movies and the popular media certainly seem to have given more attention to it. Let me now draw up a picture:

The private psychiatric hospital is a multi-turreted building. It is always on a hill and it is always—24 hours a day—covered in a murky fog. If you listen carefully as you approach it, and you must always do so from a long distance, you will probably hear Merle Oberon crying, "Heathcliff," as she looks for Laurence Olivier.

You now enter this cold, sterile building to be met by Nurse Ratched, played most appropriately by Agnes Moorehead. With a snap of her fingers, two attendants appear—Lon Chaney, Jr., and King Kong! The doctor—and there must always be a doctor—is called Dr. Uriah Heep and has to be played by John Carradine. He is accompanied by his deformed son, most likely Peter Lorre.

The patient in this myth—and there has to be a patient—is always well, not completely well, but *extremely rich*, and a white Anglo-Saxon Protestant.

The process of hospitalization in a private psychiatric hospital then becomes how fast can Dr. Heep, Nurse Ratched, and the attendants take this healthy person, denude him of all of his assets, please his family by doing so, and at the same time, have enough energy so that they can send the dogs out to look for Merle Oberon and bring her back in.

With this as prologue, we can now get into the realities of what is and what has been a private psychiatric hospital. Since we are going to talk about the last 100 years, probably the most appropriate place to begin and to center in on would be South Oaks Hospital.

It began in 1882 as a psychiatric hospital and has been in continuous operation since. One might ask, at this point, "It must be the oldest psychiatric hospital in existence and what could they possibly have done for patients in that time?" It is more important to be aware that at the time this hospital opened, McLean Hospital in Massachusetts and Friends Hospital in Philadelphia had been in operation for 60 to 70 years, and that they were young upstarts in comparison to The Institute of Pennsylvania Hospital.

The Institute began in 1751 and has been serving the public's mental health needs for 231 years. Two hundred and thirty-one years is long before the world heard of not only John Carradine and Nurse Ratched, but also 140 years before the world was even aware that there was a man named Sigmund Freud. Private mental hospitals in this country had been operating before Dorothea Dix, before Clifford Beers, and before Charcot.

A question that came to my mind after I had agreed to give this speech was, what did they do for people 100 years ago? I recently spoke to the medical director of The Brattleboro Retreat which was founded in Vermont in 1834. They are going through some of their old papers not only to find out what was done for the patients, but how the patients got there, how did people live, how, for example, did they heat hospitals, what employees did they have, etc.

As far as can be determined, there were no psychiatrists as we know them today and there were certainly none of the ancillary professions. That means that people were treated and did get well—they got well because we know that they were admitted and we know that they left the hospital and we know that they functioned and they did this without psychiatrists as we know now; certainly without psychologists for psychology had its beginnings in 1871 in Leipzig, Germany.

We know that the hospital was without recreational and occupational therapy, it was without a record room librarian, and, in fact, unbelievable as it may sound, it was without the Joint Commission on Accreditation of Hospitals.

The hospitals did have nurses, they had attendants and, most often, they had superintendents who had little or no professional training. Some of the early psychiatric hospitals were headed by farmers or businessmen or builders.

The form of treatment in the beginning did not, of course, include psychotherapy for the term was unknown and the science had not yet been worked out. It did not include chemotherapy which did not come until well along in the 20th century, it did not include electrotherapy as we know it today, and it certainly did not include psychosurgery.

An examination of our old records and those of some of the hospitals who considered us a young upstart indicate that there was tremendous emphasis on what we now know as milieu therapy. Patients who were admitted invariably came from what was then a long distance. South Oaks Hospital, which was known for many years as The Long Island Home Hotel for Nervous Invalids, catered primarily to patients from New York City. It is difficult enough it get here in 1982 by the Long Island Rail Road. It is an onerous journey by the Long Island Expressway, but imagine what it must have taken to make this long trip in the 1880's. Records indicate that our stage coach met the train twice a day. Brattleboro Retreat is near Dartmouth College, quite removed even today, and yet people would come and stay there.

Most of the early records indicate that patients were made a part of the family. They lived with the staff who lived on the grounds. They did some work and one gains the impression that a tremendous amount of human care and treatment was given. We have pictures of patients accompanied by their attendant, both carrying guns, going to the Great South Bay for a day of duck shooting. There are records that indicate that patients worked on the farm and helped with the chores. Obviously this milieu therapy approach, which was certainly long-term, brought about positive results in a great many of the patients who were treated.

We did not engage in the kind of behavior which was reported in the 1895 edition of the *American Journal of Insanity,* under the heading, "A Peripatetic Insane Asylum":

> In Elda, in the Province of Alicante, there is an insane asylum whose officials draw their pay from the treasury of the provincial deputation—or rather should do so—but, as all too often happens in lovely Spain, it is now and then the case that the officials wait for months for their salary, because the treasury stands empty.
>
> A few days ago the President of the provincial deputation remembered that for some six months there had been no remittance to the asylum. He therefore thought it advisable to send the cashier with funds to the institution. When the latter, however, arrived in Elda he found that he could not accomplish the disbursement of the salaries, for the reason that the asylum stood empty and abandoned. Not a soul was there. In the village, the cashier was informed that the officials, weary of their long waiting, had, some weeks before, in company with the mad folk, formed a musical organization and were now traversing the country, earning their bread by playing at balls and fairs. The authorities ordered the arrest of the deserters.

As far as we know, such behavior was confined to Spain.

In 1842 Charles Dickens visited what was then called The Hartford Retreat and he marvelled that:

> Every patient in this asylum sits down to dinner every day with a knife and fork, and in the midst of them sits the gentleman (butler) whose manner of dealing with the charges I have just described . . . At every meal moral influence alone re-

strains the more violent among them from cutting the throats of the rest. But the effect of that influence is reduced to an absolute certainty and is found even as a measure of restraint to say nothing of it as a means of cure, and is a hundred times more efficacious than all the strait waistcoats, fetters, and handcuffs that ignorance, prejudice, and cruelty have manufactured since the creation of the world.

These early hospitals probably did as good work as they did because they maintained a very low census. This hospital, for example, with far more than 80 acres, carried a census of six patients at times in the 1890's. There are indications of frequent visits by families and because of the number of entries of "so-and-so ran away," we can infer that security was lax and doors must have been kept open.

The impression that one gains from reading the records of the 1880's and 1890's is that the open hospital that we began to speak of in the 1960's, 70's, and 80's was a reality 100 years ago. Fees were certainly lower then in comparison to the income of families than they are today. The records, in spite of the absence of apparent sophisticated training on the part of the staff, were fairly complete. For example, in the records of 1908 at South Oaks, there is a note that a patient had expressed delusions of persecution in regard to the physicians and nurses: "She says that the medicine I have given her is meant to retard her recovery and that the milk the nurses gave her is drugged. Physically she is doing well." This patient improved to the point that the last note says, "Patient has shown so much improvement during the summer, it seemed proper to parole her and accordingly she went home today in the custody of her brother."

Private psychiatric hospitals have always been in the forefront of positive changes in the mental health field. New therapies and new approaches have come far more from the private sector than from the public. The great psychiatric hospitals of our country are the private psychiatric hospitals. The Menninger Foundation is and has always been a private hospital. Brattleboro Retreat, which has been a private hospital since 1834, also provided all the psychiatric care for the entire state of Vermont over a 60-year period. During this 60-year period which ended relatively recently, they were responsible not only for their private hospital, but they staffed and managed the state hospital. Chestnut Lodge is another of our eminent psychiatric hospitals and is also a private hospital. "I Never Promised You A Rose Garden" is the story of a patient at Chestnut Lodge and the fictional psychiatrist is based on the real-life psychiatrist, the late Freda Fromm-Reichmann. Hospitals such as Chestnut Lodge pioneered inpatient psychoanalytical long-term treatment of patients.

Other hospitals which are leaders in their field and are private psychiatric hospitals include not only The Institute of Pennsylvania Hospital, but also Sheppard & Enoch Pratt in Baltimore; McLean Hospital in Belmont, Massachusetts, which is one of the teaching hospitals of the Harvard Medical School; the Yale Psychiatric Institute in New Haven; Austen Riggs in Massachusetts where Erik Erikson and his wife are involved in first having established and then running therapy programs; and New York Hospital—Westchester Division, which has a long and distinguished record in treating patients. Modesty almost made me keep South Oaks Hospital off this list, but I have decided to include it. South Oaks, founded 100 years ago, is one of the older more eminent hospitals.

It is generally acknowledged that a relatively small group of psychiatric hospitals espoused the moral treatment of what were first called "lunatics" and then "the insane"; that these small private hospitals were instrumental in bringing patients out of the almshouses, and the attics, and the prisons. This humanitarian care of the mentally ill fortunately continued not only in the private sector but in the public sector.

There are at least a few interesting anecdotes regarding these early psychiatric hospitals. From the very beginning of the founding of this hospital, there was involvement by the state. What is now called The Office of Mental Health and was called The Department of Mental Hygiene not too many years ago, was called The State Commission in Lunacy in the 1880's. We have minutes of the Lunacy Commissioner coming to the hospital and evaluating programs. In 1886 there is a record that the State Commissioner in Lunacy advised that "mild patients are to be given even more liberty." He obviously saw himself as a union leader for he said, as far back as 1890, "The salary of an assistant physician shall be increased to at least $50 a month and he should be required to devote all of his time to the work of the institution." This same Commissioner also said attendants should be required to keep their uniforms in a tidy condition and the attendants who shave should do so when *not* on duty.

By the early 1900's the term "lunacy" had taken on a pejorative connotation and the Commission's name was changed to the State Hospital Commission.

It is fascinating to read some of these early minutes in that the things that we now take so much for granted were so new in the past. There is a record in 1890 that the hospital had installed its first telephone and it was followed a short time later by a report that the telephone was in "unworking order." That may be because the phone did not work or it may be there was no one to call. In any event, in 1891 the minutes record that, "on motion the secretary was directed to notify the company to put the machine in good working order or take it out."

The field of psychiatric hospitals has made positive

strides in a relatively short time. We must keep in mind when we talk about private psychiatric hospitals that it is really a very small group. The National Association of Private Psychiatric Hospitals (NAPPH), which is the national organization for free-standing hospitals, was organized but 50 years ago and has but 201 members. There are a total in the 50 states of only 23,000 beds in private psychiatric hospitals where most of the advances have taken place. If we add the combined total of all the other psychiatric beds in general hospitals' psychiatric divisions, there are only 24,000 more—a total of only 47,000 beds for all.

With the fact that on Long Island not too long ago Pilgrim State Hospital had 18,000 patients, Central Islip had 15,000, Kings Park in the neighborhood of 12,000, and Creedmoor about 8,000, that means that in a distance of perhaps 50 miles, there were more psychiatric patients in state hospitals than there are private psychiatric hospital beds in the entire nation. It is amazing that the relatively small group of private psychiatric hospitals and small group of patients have produced the results in the quality of care that they have.

Private psychiatric hospitals accounted for only 3 percent of the total patient care episode in 1975. In all likelihood they probably never provided more than 5 percent of that care and yet they have continued to be a major force in providing mental health services. In 1948, Albert Deutsch, who wrote "The Shame of the States" in which he expressed his thesis that the mentally ill deserved more than the custodial warehousing and neglect to which they were then relegated, described private psychiatric hospitals in a far more favorable manner. He spoke of certain private psychiatric hospitals as being engaged in major programs of research. He saw them as free-standing accredited training centers in affiliation with academic centers. He expressed the belief that many private psychiatric hospitals offered physicians an opportunity to learn from intensive work with a small number of patients under the tutelage of experienced clinicians: He saw private psychiatric hospitals as models of excellence committed to serving the patient which, again in a comparison with the other types of treatment in this country, is probably a very valid appraisal.

As a sample of the kind of contributions that a small private hospital can make, let me tell you something about South Oaks. This is a hospital licensed for only 280 patients and it provides training via university affiliations with the Medical School of Stony Brook University, Adelphi University, Tufts University, Columbia University, and New York University. We involve ourselves with the training of resident physicians and doctoral students in clinical psychology. We have an internship program in clinical psychology; we train psychiatric nurses; we train occupational therapists and recreational therapists and social workers. We do this with relatively little fanfare as do most private psychiatric hospitals.

We constantly hear inquiries or rhetorical questions as to whether or not there is more mental illness today than there was in the past and answers that range from, "There must be," to "No, it is now more recognized." From a statistical standpoint we know that patient care episodes more than quadrupled between 1955 and 1975. In 1955 there were 1.7 million episodes and in 1975 there were 6.9 million. The rate of patient care episodes per 100,000 population tripled, increasing from 1,000 in 1955 to 3,000 in 1975. Inpatient episodes accounted for 77 percent of the total in 1955, but only 27 percent of the total by 1975, with 70 percent outpatients.

If one is to understand what it is that a private psychiatric hospital does, we should talk about staff/patient ratios. In 1974 there were 204 total staff members for every 100 patients in private hospitals. In state and county mental hospitals the number was only 88. Obviously if you have a staff that is more than 200 percent higher, you are able to provide a quality of care that is unavailable with the smaller staff and you are able to do it in a shorter time.

A statement such as that inevitably brings forth some comments such as, "Of course if you have a great deal of money and spend a great deal of money, you can get better care. What happens to those people who cannot afford care?" A more germane question might be, "How much does it cost in comparison to a public psychiatric hospital?" A reasonable basis of comparison would be the cost of a private hospital with the cost of an acute care unit such as at Nassau County Medical Center. If you carefully compare the rates of the private psychiatric hospitals with the rates of the public institutions, you will surprisingly find that the cost of public hospitalization is far greater than that of the private hospital. If you compare the costs of a free-standing psychiatric hospital with a general hospital's psychiatric division, you will most often find that the cost of the general hospital far exceeds the free-standing psychiatric hospital. That should do much to blot out the myth of phenomenally high costs.

There has to be a reason why the costs are lower. Part of it is obvious and it really represents the difference between private enterprise and public projects. Private enterprise must be more responsive to the marketplace and, because it does not have a cumbersome bureaucracy, it is able to move much more rapidly. Moreover, in comparison to a general hospital, private hospitals save a great deal of money for the patients. For example, it does not have to have a fully-staffed operating room or an operating room at all. It does not have to have a CAT scan, a hyperbaric chamber, and so forth. In many of the less populated states, there is a move away from the state hospital, which has proven so expensive and cumbersome, to subsidizing care in private hospitals where the care is better, the length of stay shorter, and the costs lower.

Because of this need to compete in the marketplace for patients, private hospitals have striven for excellence that goes beyond simply meeting the needs of an acceptable level of quality. The need to please the consumer, which is emerging in recent years as an almost novel concept, has been a part of the private psychiatric hospital for all of its existence. The main purpose of private psychiatric hospitals is to serve the patient. As a result, they have come to serve as models against which other programs are measured. We must also keep in mind that treating the mentally ill is not only one of several services as it is in a general hospital, but it is the *reason for being* in a free-standing psychiatric hospital. If the needs of the psychiatric patient are not met, the hospital fails.

Continuing on with the thesis that the free enterprise system is the one that works best, it is the ability of private hospitals to go out into the marketplace to hire the best talent that aids in providing the quality of service that it does. Leaders in the mental health field frequently come from the private sector. Over just the last 11 years, for example, and from a group of only 201 hospitals with just 23,000 beds, there have been three people who have been presidents of the American Psychiatric Association. Considering the relatively small number of psychiatrists affiliated with private psychiatric hospitals, this goes far beyond statistical expectation. Over the past 11 years, A.P.A. presidents have been Dr. Talkington from Timberlawn Hospital in Dallas, Dr. Garber from The Carrier Clinic, and Dr. Gibson from Sheppard & Enoch Pratt.

These men have also served as presidents of the National Association of Private Psychiatric Hospitals. Two members of this hospital serve with the NAPPH. Dr. Carone is the First Vice President and should become President in 1984, and I am on the Long-Range Planning Committee and the Program Committee.

As one looks at a small rather unheralded hospital such as South Oaks, some idea as to excellence of staff and its connection with quality of care becomes evident. We have a staff of 16 psychiatrists, four psychologists, four social workers, six registered occupational therapists and eight recreational specialists for a patient population of approximately 250.

Fourteen of the psychiatrists are board certified in psychiatry and the other two are board eligible. Two of our psychologists are board certified in clinical psychology by the American Board of Professional Psychology and three of our social workers are members of the Academy of Certified Social Workers. We have 71 registered nurses, 34 with a Bachelor of Science degree and six with a Master of Science degree. Our occupational therapists are licensed by the New York State Education Department.

When a small hospital can field such an array of talent, we begin to get a somewhat better idea as to why there is so much psychotherapy, why patients are seen daily, and why lengths of stay are shorter. While costs are relatively high, the overall cost is less than it would be in a public acute-care hospital. Add to this that we have a staff to patient ratio of far better than two to one, and this understanding of what happens in a private hospital becomes even clearer.

The private psychiatric hospital field has not only spawned leaders of professional organizations, but it has also been in the forefront of the move toward delivery of quality care. The mission of the private free-standing psychiatric hospital is to promote high quality care and treatment for the psychiatrically ill and to do so in as cost-effective and efficient a manner as is possible.

The National Association of Private Psychiatric Hospitals was one of the founding sponsors of The Accreditation Council for Psychiatric Facilities for The Joint Commission on Accreditation of Hospitals. Many of the surveyors whom we have personally met and whom we know have had careers in private hospitals as nurses, psychiatrists, psychologists, and social workers before taking on the surveying job. While there is an increasing number of surveyors who are now doing this on a full-time basis, many of the other surveyors are retired professionals from the private sectors who are involved on a part-time basis.

There are weaknesses in the private sector and while it is hoped that the strengths compensate for these, the weaknesses are present. Because of the relatively small number of hospitals and because they tend to be centered in large metropolitan areas, there are vast areas where such quality care for the psychiatrically ill patient is unavailable. As it always means in such cases, the public sector must step in because the private sector finds that it is not an advantageous place for them to be.

While the private hospitals have had an effect on the delivery of services, the group as a whole and each individual hospital are really too small to have other than a minimal impact. Some of the weaknesses have been most evident in recent years as the scope of the mental health field has expanded. There has been increasing community involvement. The hospitals are trying to do everything for everyone and the staff is spread too thin. This often results in an overly diffused focus.

Another weakness is that the hospitals have a very loose confederation, basically only their association with The National Association of Private Psychiatric Hospitals. The result is that they are often unable to inform the public about what they do. This inability to reach the consumer results in consumers being willing to accept a mediocre level of care that they might not accept if they had a real understanding of what is involved in quality care. This weakness takes us back to the first parts of this presentation in which I pointed out that, amongst other things, it is the Hollywood version of what a psychiatric hospital is, as compared to the reality of it, that dictates the public's expectations.

What are the *strengths* of the hospital? The goal of each psychiatric hospital is a unified one, namely, to provide care solely for psychiatric patients. While the small size often causes certain problems, it is this same relatively small size that tends to insure a personal approach and quality care. It is the small size and the absence of a major bureaucracy that allows the private hospital to adapt quickly to changing conditions and to institute new programs.

As an example, in a hospital such as South Oaks, as we anticipated the need, we moved into a drug abuse program, an alcoholism program, a program for substance-abusing acting-out adolescents and an adolescent program for emotionally disturbed young people. Our Board of Cooperative Educational Services junior-senior high school program dates back to the very beginning of the adolescent program. By virtue of our size and the fact that the administration is not a part of a large bureaucracy, we can make decisions, get the support of the governing body, and be in operation long before other larger, more cumbersome institutions. This also permits us to change direction to meet the needs of the public and to drop programs when they are no longer needed. Our experience has been that it is this ability to add as well as to drop programs that is a principal strength.

A prime example of being able to institute new programs is in what we're doing at this twelfth South Oaks Hospital/Stony Brook University Conference on Industrial Psychiatric Medicine. In the early 1970's we recognized a need to involve industry more completely in the mental health process. We saw the need for a coalition between industry and hospitals. It was about the same time that we also saw a need to involve the clergy more meaningfully than they had been. Within several months we organized our first conference on "Alcoholism in Industry" and followed this with others such as "Drug Abuse in Industry," "Women in Industry," and "Misfits in Industry." In the same period we instituted our annual Clergy and Mental Health Conferences with topics such as "Alienation, Loneliness, and Depression as Seen by the Clergy and Mental Health Professionals," "Family Counseling and Therapy—The Role of the Clergy and Mental Health Professionals," and "Mid-Life Crisis: Where Have I Been? Where Am I Going?"

In line with our awareness of the need to involve industry, we established a number of contacts with both labor and management. We began to serve as consultants to both groups and the result is that increasing numbers of people who need care have since been receiving it in a cost-effective fashion.

Strength is seen in the private hospitals' willingness to offer a wide variety of care both in and outside the hospital. More and more the private hospital is offering outpatient care and aftercare services, maintaining its commitment to quality care. It has established relationships with other health institutions via transfer agreements. On a more concrete level, the result is that all of the South Oaks psychiatrists maintain affiliations and serve in a consultant capacity to a number of general hospitals and their psychiatric divisions. We provide the same consultant relationships to a number of nursing homes with the care of their geriatric patients and are also of aid to serve self-help organizations for adolescents.

Another factor that should be seen as a strength is the stability of the private hospital. All of us who have lived in the Long Island area know about the effects of de-institutionalization. The state hospitals are emptying and there has been a question for a number of years as to which ones will close.

The private hospital recognizes that de-institutionalization has certain values but perhaps even more dangers. We are committed to remaining in operation and to meeting the psychiatric needs of those who need help. In this respect, and to conclude this presentation, I quote from the first Minutes of our hospital, as stated in March 1881:

> The need of an institution, such a one as the title indicates and especially designed for the treatment, care and cure of the masses of the many nervous invalids, and upon pecuniary terms of easy access to them personally and their friends, who may propose to patronize the Home Hotel, being unanimously conceded, not only as a county and state necessity but also as urgent benevolent enterprise, it was resolved, forthwith to organize by the election of Trustees . . .

It is a statement that applies to South Oaks and to most of the prestigious private psychiatric hospitals in the country.

Question-and-Answer Session

Audience:
Private hospitals are often criticized for either not taking indigent patients or for moving patients to state facilities as soon as the money runs out. In your research, did you gather any data on the commitment of private hospitals to the care of patients who can't pay?

Dr. Krinsky:
I didn't gather data on other hospitals, but I can tell you what we do. We have some long-term patients, and we

have a commitment to these patients. At the present time we have arranged, via our Board of Directors, for a special fee for these patients that is so low that you probably couldn't stay in a boarding house for that amount of money. We also have had patients who have, at certain points, run out of money. Because of our short length of stay now—30 to 32 days—if that happens, we keep the patient. We do not send patients out who are ill. The myth of "Wait until we get the last dollar and shove them out" is simply untrue. My experience with other private psychiatric hospitals is that, by and large, they do the same thing.

Audience:

You made the comment that quality care makes a difference. Do you know of studies, that prove, for example, that the treatment of schizophrenia would be better if it were evaluated carefully under quality care than under other kinds of care such as that given by a state hospital?

Dr. Krinsky:

No, but I'm sure that studies are being done. It would just seem that it would be self-evident. The private psychiatric hospital with a short length of stay and what appears to be comparable or better results than longer lengths of stay in other hospitals would certainly seem to be one of the criteria that we would use as a measurement.

Audience:

Do private psychiatric hospitals ever give out any free beds on admission?

Dr. Krinsky:

Recognizing the needs of our community, we have given 2,265 patient days per year to a number of agencies in this area. Among the recipients of our free beds are the

State University of New York at Stony Brook, and the Long Island Council on Alcoholism. What this means is that if someone is indigent and needs care, there is no charge for any of the services we provide up to the number of patient free days that we have allotted. We have always offered more free days than have been used by any of the organizations to whom we have given them, so obviously, it's a large number.

Audience:
I'd much rather be in a private hospital than in any state institution. The surroundings alone are conducive to getting better. And even if you don't get better quickly, at least you're in a nice place. Do you take any people who are life-long patients, the chronic schizophrenic, or the chronic paranoid, or do you take any forensic cases which are sent in by the courts?

Dr. Krinsky:
We will take all of those. However, one of the things that we have found is that symptoms seem to have changed in mental illness over the last years. We accept the idea that symptoms are really reflective of a patient's cry for need, cry for help. If you think back many years ago, you had hysterical paralysis. That was followed by waxy flexibility, acute catatonic acting-out. Now you don't see those any longer. I think that as people are becoming much more attuned to illness—we're probably living in the age of depression now—we are seeing the acutely ill patient; those are the poeple who are turning to us for service. The scope of our treatment program is geared for a medium-term acute care, as our median length of stay is 30 to 32 days. By process of elimination, we are not seeing the long-term chronic patients any longer. We will admit forensic cases, but again, one of the advantages of being a private hospital is that you

can choose the kind of patients that you best treat. A hospital has never claimed that it is all things to all people. If there are forensic cases that we can handle well and within our length of stay, we will take such a patient.

Audience:
How do you deal with the courts?

Dr. Krinsky:
When we deal with a court we clearly state our policy, pointing out that if they wish to send a patient here, the patient must fit into the general mainstream of our patient population. No private hospital is big enough to provide all the multiple units that a state institution does. However, the quality of service is infinitely better.

Chapter 6

THE PUBLIC MENTAL HOSPITAL— THE LAST 100 YEARS

Walter E. Barton, M.D.*

The centennial of South Oaks Hospital is a joyous celebration of achievement and an opportunity to review the history of mental hospitals during the past 100 years. Founded under the laws of the State of New York in 1881, South Oaks Hospital—which was then known as The Long Island Home Hotel for Nervous Invalids—received its first patients in its main building in 1882.

One hundred years ago in 1882:[1]

---

*Walter E. Barton, M.D., is an active Professor of Psychiatry (Emeritus) at the Dartmouth Medical School. His career spans over half of the last 100 years, in part at Worcester State Hospital (1931–1942) and Boston State Hospital (1945–1963) where he served as Superintendent. Dr. Barton is a Past President and Past Medical Director of the American Psychiatric Association, and has served as President of the American Board of Psychiatry and Neurology, the Group for Advancement of Psychiatry, and the American College of Mental Health Administration, among others.

- Tchaikovsky's "1812 Overature," Wagner's "Parsi-fal" and Gilbert and Sullivan's "Iolanthe" were composed.
- Cezanne and Monet were acclaimed for new paintings.
- Robert L. Stevenson wrote "Treasure Island."
- Queen Victoria and John L. Sullivan reigned.
- F.D.R. was born and Charles Darwin died.
- The Fenian's (forerunners of the IRA) murdered Lord Frederick Cavendish and T. H. Burke in a park in Dublin, Ireland.
- The assassin, Charles Guiteau, who shot President James Garfield, was hanged in Washington, D.C.
- Dorothea Dix, who had retired the year before, was living at the Trenton State Hospital, having completed 40 years of unparalleled work building mental hospitals and improving conditions for the mentally ill.
- Joseph Breuer, in Vienna, used hypnosis to treat hysteria.
- The first nurses' training in a mental hospital was inaugurated at McLean Hospital.

Mental Hospitals

The small highly successful public asylum of the moral treatment era had passed. The standard that had been set by the Association of Medical Superintendents of American Institutions for the Insane (now the American Psychiatric Association), limiting the size of asylums to 250 beds, had been broken. In New York, Utica State Hospital had 600 patients and Willard State Hospital had 1,200. The factors of population pressure, chronicity, relationship to welfare issues, and indigency responsible for the increasing numbers of mentally ill individuals were known as a consequence of the widely disseminated and discussed findings of the Jarvis report.[2]

Moral treatment succeeded when individual attention to patients was possible in small hospitals and when staff shared values of the Protestant native-born, middle-class patients. Wave upon wave of immigrants washed upon the shores of the new country. At best, adjustment to the new culture was fragile for the impoverished family. Extrusion of an insane member to care in an institution could mean survival for the rest of the family who could not afford to cease work to provide care. Society was reluctant to spend huge sums of money to build new hospitals or new buildings and to pay for care of "foreigners." The insane, from another culture seemed less responsive to moral treatment, and illness became chronic. The resentment against increasing taxes led to underfinancing and understaffing of public institutions.[3]

To handle the ever increasing new admissions and accumulating chronic patients, some institutions limited admission to bed capacity with no room for acute cases. Others sent the chronically ill to almshouses where the county became responsible for care. The consequence of enforced economy was substandard custodial care.

In spite of Edward Jarvis's recommendations to the contrary,[2] Massachusetts set up Gardner and Grafton State Hospitals to house chronic patients. Soon there was enough community pressure to admit acute cases.

Social policy dictated that all patients who could work were to do so and contribute labor to reduce costs. Farm colonies were an extension of the mental hospital and patients worked on the farm or in all institution support services.

In 1884 Daniel Tuke visited the United States. In comparison with care in Great Britain, he noted excessive reliance on restraint and seclusion, a lack of research (except at McLean) and a lack of emphasis upon scientific clinical care. He found wards barren, bleak, and unfurnished. Tuke lauded the finding of more physicians on the staff of mental hospitals in the United States and salaries higher than in England. Tuke believed they overemphasized efficiency and administrative matters to the neglect of clinical tasks.[4]

A survey, "Lunacy in Many Lands," made in 1885 by an Australian, George Tucker, noted the reprehensible use of cages, iron chains, handcuffs, straps, crib-beds and chairs screwed to the floor. He deplored the lack of occupation and diversion. Tucker did find some exceptions and cited Danvers (Massachusetts) where wards were pleasantly furnished with pictures, flowers, and singing birds. Their aides wore aprons and caps, and actually attended patients, not only on acute wards but also on chronic wards.

Other assessments of care in the 1890's[4,5,6] found patients stripped of possessions and dignity, desocialized, degraded, living in well-regulated hopelessness. Inmates lived in dormitory barracks, bathed once weekly in open basement areas, had no privacy in doorless rows of toilets that had no seat covers. Treatment reflected the state of the art: sedatives, purgatives, and tonics, with restraint and seclusion for the unruly. Those who could, worked. A social hour in the evening might feature a magic lantern slide show. Records were minimally kept in a bound case book that served all admitted.

In 1884, on the occasion of the 40th anniversary of the founding of the Association of Medical Superintendents, there were 44,000 patients in 130 institutions. The association had grown to 115 members. Three of the founders were still alive, Kirkbride, Earle, and Butler. At the annual meeting the vexing problem of restraint was again addressed noting that calamitous accidents occurred when not used. Attention was directed to the need for color, draperies and furnishings for wards. Attendants were to become companions of patients, not keepers.

The currents of reform reflected an optimistic moralism. If a problem was defined, a solution could be found. Traditional assumptions were re-examined in the search for ways to improve care. The models to be followed were Hartford Retreat and McLean, private mental hospitals caring for the middle and upper classes and not the population silting-up the public mental hospitals.

It was at a state hospital in Worcester, Massachusetts, once the national model, that had deteriorated under the pressures of problems shared by all state institutions, that a young physician, Adolf Meyer began, in 1898, his teaching career that would influence the system and its practitioners for the next 40 years. Meyer viewed the human organism as dynamic, reacting and transforming its environment and being influenced by it. He taught the science of observation and the study of the living. To get a complete history he utilized what became psychiatric social workers to evaluate home and work environment. Individual clinical records were developed and continuing education was implemented to update knowledge and skills. The hospital became a training center affiliated with Clark University, whose faculty assisted in teaching physicians while Meyer taught psychologists. A laboratory was established at the hospital to study the brain and all physicians were involved in the studies, integrating clinical and research endeavors. To relieve the burden upon physicians of manufacture of drugs, a pharmacist was hired as well as a secretary to assist with administrative tasks.

In 1887, John Butler's book "Curability of Insanity" was published. It stated that large hospitals harm patients by treating them like a mob and by denying personal attention.

In 1892, under Dr. O. J. Wilsey as superintendent, the

Long Island Home added two wings to the main building and built a laboratory. Fifty acres of land were added to the original fourteen. Expansion continued with the erection of a cottage (The Villa, 1895), a bath house/gymnasium, and connection with the village water supply (1896), all buildings were wired for electricity (1897), cottages were added in 1900 and 1903, electrical therapy and hydrotherapy rooms were opened and sun parlors were built on the main buildings (1904).

S. Weir Mitchell, the country's most distinguished neurologist, who was also a novelist, poet, and contributor to the scientific literature which included his widely known "rest cure" (in "Fat and Blood, and How to Make Them," J. B. Lippincott Co., 1877) was invited to address the 1894 meeting of the American Psychiatric Association which was then called the American Medico-Psychological Association. He castigated the physicians present for their professional isolation from the rest of medicine, for their lack of research, and for their lack of application of new knowledge. Receptive to the deserved criticism, his message served as a catalyst to corrective action.

The First Two Decades of the 20th Century

Of the many streams which impinged upon mental hospitals to change them in the first 20 years of the new century, I have elected to note only four: Freud's creative insights, a prophetic experiment at the Peoria State Hospital, the mental hygiene movement, and the establishment of psychopathic hospitals.

Freud's "Interpretation of Dreams" (1900), "Psychopathology of Everyday Life" (1914), and "Introduction to Psychoanalysis" (1920) provided the substance for a dominant theory that was to profoundly affect psychiatry, art, history, and change social values. Freud's appearance at Clark University in 1910 was to ignite the fire that spread his ideas in the United States aided by the support of James J. Putnam, A. A. Brill, and William A. White and Ernest Jones in Canada.

The winds of change went almost unnoticed in 1905 when McFarland and Zeller conducted a demonstration of prophetic insight into the future of the mental hospital. At the Peoria State Hospital (Illinois) they abolished all restraint, removed all iron gratings from windows, and unlocked the ward doors. Women aides worked on male wards and the eight-hour work day was instituted. Within three years the experiment was forced to end by professional contemporaries and public opinion citing two suicides as evidence that their approach was unworkable.

It would take nearly 50 years before studies would show an open hospital system did not increase the prevalence of suicide when accompanied by intensive treatment.

Clifford Beer's book "The Mind That Found Itself" (1910), an autobiographical account of experience as a patient in a mental hospital, told of neglect, dehumanization, and brutality that was to catalyze a reform effort with the aid of the National Association for Mental Hygiene of which Beers was a founder. The mental hygiene movement was second only to Dorothea Dix's work on behalf of the mentally ill. Improved clinical care, increased fiscal support and research were objectives of the citizen organization aided by leaders in the mental hospital field.

A new kind of mental hospital, well staffed, small in beds, was established in Albany (1906), Ann Arbor (1906), Toronto (1908) and by the Boston State Hospital (1912). The psychopathic hospital was to be the general hospital for mental disorders bringing together clinical care, teaching and research. The new organization quickly demonstrated its superiority to large public mental hospitals and became the sought-after place to secure training.

World War I was to contribute valuable insights to patient care in civilian hospitals as well as in the military. Thomas Salmon noted that:

- Stress (combat) produced mental illness.
- Therapist attitudes influenced outcome.
- Early treatment (in forward areas in combat zones) reduced disability.
- Rest, food, assurance and support, suggestions and ventilation of feelings were the basis for treatment.

In public mental hospitals, case loads increased as did the numbers of chronically ill. Care was often custodial and at best compassionate and supportive.

Administrative issues featured in presentations to the 75th annual meeting of the APA (1919) advocated were:

- A central agency for state hospital management.
- Adherence to Kirkbride construction standards:
  Placement in less stressful environment, outskirts of town, farms and gardens with work opportunity and recreation in clean wholesome wards.
- Psychopathic hospital development.

The Revolution in Treatment 1920–1940

The general hospital unit for psychiatric patients was not new. The Pennsylvania Hospital had pioneered such a unit in 1753 but growth was almost imperceptible until Henry Ford Hospital (Detroit) opened such a unit in 1924 and others followed with a surge of new units in the 1930's.

It was the development of new therapies which speeded the change in the delivery system. All of the therapies developed out of practice and experience in mental hospitals. Hydrotherapy introduced by Dent in 1902, who cited the work of Simon Baruch, spread widely under development and promotion by Rebecca Wright. Continuous tubs and wet sheet packs were sedative agents for excitement and hot and cold sprays stimulating. All mental hospitals developed hydrotherapy units.

In 1922 the focal infection theory of causation of "autointoxication" under Cotton led to a search for possible sources of infection with the gastro-intestinal tract, teeth and tonsils likely sources and so surgical correction was undertaken. Colonic irrigations became a standard technique for removing potential pollutants from the body. Its use persisted into the 1930's when I was a resident at Worcester State Hospital and learned the technique.

In 1918, Wagner Von Jauregg in Vienna discovered the treponema pallidum. Later it was learned heat destroyed the germ that caused central nervous system syphilis which was responsible for about 12 percent of public mental hospital admissions. St. Elizabeths Hospital in Washington, D.C., was the source for the strain of malaria used by mental hospitals to induce fever in patients with syphilis. In Worcester, we used diathermy to generate heat.

Goldfarb and Spies discovered the cure for pellagra (diarrhea, dementia and death) in 1928 and another mental illness became preventable and disappeared from admissions.

In 1933 Sakel (Austria) introduced insulin as a treatment for schizophrenia. D. Ewen Cameron and Roy Hoskins at Worcester State Hospital established one of the first units for insulin therapy in this country. Two years later Von Meduna (Budapest) used injected metrazal to induce convulsions to treat schizophrenia. It was promptly widely utilized. Moniz in Lisbon (1935) developed prefrontal lobotomy. Because this therapy severed connecting fibers in the brain and required a neurosurgeon and a trained surgical team, it was slower to develop. It was not until post-World War II that experimental trials demonstrated its benefit in selected cases. Walter Freeman, a psychiatrist, developed an "ice pick" operative procedure with supraorbital insertion. Opposition to multilative procedures on the brain was intense enough to curtail its use and it continues to be an experimental therapy in the 1980's.

It was Cerletti and Bini's (Italy) introduction of Electric Convulsive Therapy (ECT) in 1938 that began a treatment so remarkable in its prompt relief of symptoms that it was responsible in large part for a revolution in the system of delivery of care for mental disorders. Lothar Kalinowsky in New York, Meyerson in Boston, and Neyman in Chicago, were pioneers in its application. All mental hospitals used the treatment first in excited schizophrenics and agitated depressions and later in various forms of depressive disorders. For the first time a series of 10 treatments over a few weeks caused a dramatic remission in symptoms. Patients who formerly stayed months in a hospital could be successfully treated in a matter of days. E.C.T. units were developed in general hospitals. Some private hospitals were opened with E.C.T. the principle therapy and a few psychiatrists gave the therapy in their offices.

Abraham Meyerson (1939) at Boston State Hospital instituted a forerunner of what was to become milieu therapy. To combat the dependency, loss of initiative, and deterioration which has been called "institutional neurosis" (the consequences of custodial care), Meyerson introduced what he called "total push therapy." He marshalled all hospital resources to design an individual program of scheduled activities to foster relationships that, when coupled with staff attitudes of encouragement with interaction with patients, resulted in improvement.

Other events in the period 1920–1940 worth noting were:

- The first day hospital at Adams Nervine (Boston) which made a full day of treatment possible without becoming an inpatient.
- The development of a relationship between religion and psychiatry which led to pastoral counseling at Worcester State Hospital (Anton Boisson, 1933).
- A remarkable demonstration of public mental hospital improved patient care was made possible at Worcester by the Great Depression. It became possible to employ the best psychiatrists and nurses to entend therapy and group activities.
- William A. Bryan's pioneering book "Administrative Psychiatry," a benchmark for literature in the field, and for public mental hospital improvement.

The Decline of Mental Hospitals and the Beginning of the Revolution in the Delivery of Mental Health Services 1940–1960

Although experience had revealed one in four casualties would be a psychiatric disorder, the military was unprepared when World War II began. The recorded experience of World War I was forgotten. Out of the global war, once again, important lessons were learned with application to civilian mental hospital practice and to the delivery of services. Some of them were:

- The mental hygiene consultation service model.
- Outpatient management of psychiatric disorders.
- Physical medicine rehabilitation services.
- Crises intervention and group therapy.
- Multidisciplinary team approaches.

When psychiatric casualties were promptly cared for in the combat zone, 20 percent to 40 percent of those with combat neuroses returned to full combat duty, and 40 percent to 60 percent to full non-combat duty. Noted also were the salutory effects of early ambulation after surgery, early return to units, replacements as a group rather than as individuals as survival depended upon group response, and confirmation of the statement "everyone has a breaking point under stress."

The policy of the Veterans Administration to include a psychiatric unit in every V.A. general hospital accelerated the growth of general hospital psychiatry and helped make the unit the primary site for hospitalization for a mental disorder. V.A. research studies demonstrated that the Haun-type V.A. hospital (smaller, and better staffed) outperformed traditional V.A. neuropsychiatric hospitals. They were more cost effective and had a more favorable patient outcome.

Two events in 1946 made a response possible to the demand for reform in mental hospital care. The National Mental Health Act created the National Institute of Mental Health with its threefold mission to develop clinical services, manpower and training, and research. The "Young Turks," fired-up to correct deficiencies in the psychiatric field, founded the Group for the Advancement of Psychiatry. An early objective of the group was revitalization of the American Psychiatric Association. Seventeen of the next 21 APA presidents were original GAP members.

The devastation of public mental hospitals, largely due

to depletion of professional staffs during World War II, was made clear in Albert Deutsch's picture news stories and in his book "The Shame of the States," (1948).[7] It recounted the horrible conditions: no psychiatrists, lack of professional staff, overconcentration of patients, nudity and neglect.

Under the leadership of Daniel Blain, APA's first medical director and with a central headquarters staff, the first Mental Hospital Institute[8] was held in 1949 and the journal "Mental Hospitals" started as was a section on Mental Hospitals at the APA annual meeting. The focus on deficiencies and their correction, with awards given to innovative programs, did much to stimulate improvement in public mental hospitals. A Central Inspection Board made surveys of individual hospitals and an Architectural Project recommended improved facility design. Standards were formulated and applied. Studies of the English system's therapeutic community (Maxwell Jones at Belmont 1949), the open hospital (T. P. Reese and R. K. Freudenberg at Netherne), informal admissions (Duncan MacMillan at Mapperly) and a community care system (Graylingwell, J. Carse) were described in "Impressions of European Psychiatry".[9] Home visits and emergency services (A. Querido and J. H. Gravenstein's Municipal Medical and Health Services in Amsterdam) were studied and copied. The patient paid-labor program with factory-in-hospital products was applied first in V.A. Hospitals in the United States. Family Care (Zijlstra at Beilen), combined with a day treatment center and sheltered shops, provided models that were incorporated into practice in the United States as was the Soviet system for emergency care.

The unit plan in Iowa and the zone plan in Illinois related patients in public mental hospitals to their home communities and regionalized care. The Saskatchewan plan of small regional psychiatric units in community hospitals demonstrated, in 4,500 admissions, that no patient was sent to a public mental hospital. Only one of two mental hospitals became necessary in support of the system with a greatly reduced number of beds.

The Decades of Social Change and Deinstitutionalization 1960–1980

A major new direction in service delivery followed the final report "Action for Mental Health" (1961) of the Joint Commission on Mental Illness and Health. Under the leadership of APA and the National Association for Mental Health, the Community Mental Health Movement was launched. The National Institute of Mental Health provided the resources to mental hospitals under HIP (Hospital Improvement Program) grants to evaluate outreach, emergency service, transitional placements and rehabilitation. With President Kennedy's challenge to forge a new system of delivery, the Community Mental Health Center program was launched. It developed a new system of care out of the synthesis of experience in European and American mental hospitals.

The Worcester State Hospital, again in the forefront, set about to evaluate every patient in residence for placement in the community. It succeeded in reducing its census dramatically. Census in mental hospitals began to decline from administrative changes (informal and voluntary admissions, milieu therapy, open doors, paid employment) and from shift in philosophy (community care can be superior to prolonged hospital care).

The general availability of chlorpromazine (Thorazine) beginning in 1955 accelerated the decline in mental hospital census. It now became possible to treat patients with schizophrenia in the general hospital psychiatric unit or on a ambulatory basis. A whole series of anti-psychotic, anti-depressant, and anti-anxiety drugs were developed with increasing specificity in symptom relief. Deinstitutionalization was now feasible.

These trends were well underway before the social upheaval of the 1960's with the struggle of blacks and other minorities for equality. The unrest spread to college students for a greater participation in decisions concerning their education to others in protest against the war in Vietnam. The revolt against perceived social injustices was accompanied by an epidemic of drug abuse—and attitudes opposing all authority and authority in institutions. These feelings attached to mental hospitals and were expressed in anti-psychiatry. The demand for civil rights extended to rights of patients and to voiced intent to close all public mental hospitals.

The friction at the interface with the new activist law was expressed as patient rights versus patient needs.

As we begin the 100 years, 1982 and beyond, we note only a handful of public mental hospitals have closed. However, the number of patients occupying beds has dramatically dropped while patient admissions have increased and all patient encounters have expanded enormously. Boston State Hospital's census declined 87 percent in the period 1960–1980. Deinstitutionalization was possible because of:

1. Administrative reform (informal and voluntary admissions, patient responsibility for self care, work programs and open hospitals, and transitional living arrangements).
2. Conceptual shift (long stay in mental hospital is harmful, undesirable, and unneccessary; residence in the community is preferable).
3. New technology (E.C.T. and drug therapy).

4. Legal regulation (admission restricted to danger-ousness to self and others).

We pause to reflect on what mental hospitals did well and what they did poorly. What they did well:[10]

- Reflect the state of the art of medicine and social values.
- Assisted patients to develop social competence with ability to work, to utilize social skills, to accept responsibility for self care, to live outside of hospital (support in transitional facilities and in aftercare).
- Demonstrated treatability of mental disorders.
- Evaluated results of therapy.
- Developed the alternative system of care.
- Revolutionized the delivery system.

What they did poorly:

- Insufficient resources to carry out assigned mission (failure often the result of social policy beyond their control).
- Exploitation of patients "slave labor" in institutional support (change in social attitude).
- Emphasized protection of society from social dis-ruption and deviance, depriving individuals of free-dom.
- Lacked competent psychiatrists, mental health professionals and trained administrators.
- Poor personnel practices, low wages, high turnover, poorly trained aides.
- Dehumanized long-stay patients making them pow-erless and dependent.

- High proportion of involuntary admission with one-half of patients untreated.
- Confusion of goals (indigent, aged, adolescent alcohol and drugs, acute treatment, chronic care, rehabilitation of handicapped).
- Poor administration by well-intentioned clinicians.

The backlash of feeling against deinstitutionalization is strong and expressed as abandonment and neglect of the chronic mental patient in the welfare systems and in the community. The intent to close mental hospitals has changed to recognition of their continued need as a back-up to the community mental health centers to the welfare and criminal justice systems. The ambulatory care of mental disorders with brief periods of hospitalization in a general hospital is the primary care system in the 1980's. The concern over a two-tiered system (non-medical CMHC) and medical system (in office, general hospital and private mental hospital) is an unsolved issue. The medical system is growing faster than the non-medical.

The challenge of the 1980's may be summarized in the following statements:

- There is need for innovative demonstration programs in public mental hospitals of psychogeriatric units.
- Development of outreach teams to provide consultation to welfare facilities and training for caretakers.
- Effective after-care programs to insure treatment compliance and to reduce readmissions.
- Evaluation of outcome and cost effectiveness of alternative modes of care.
- Renovation of obsolete wards to reflect new function.

The economic recession of the 1980's is a time to test priorities in activities and to determine what treatment program truly makes a difference.

References

1. Grun, B.: *The Timetables of History*, Simon and Schuster, New York, 1975.
2. Jarvis, E.: *Insanity and Idiocy in Massachusetts*. Report of the Commission on Lunacy, 1855 Harvard University Press, Cambridge, 1971.
3. Deutsch, A.: *The Mentally Ill in America*, Doubleday, Doran, New York, 1937.
4. Hall, J.K., Zilboorg, G., Bunker, H.A.: *One Hundred Years of American Psychiatry*, Columbia University Press, New York, 1944.
5. Grob, G.N.: *Mental Institutions in America*, The Free Press, New York, 1973.
6. Grob, G.N.: *The State and the Mentally Ill*, University of North Carolina Press, Chapel Hill, 1966.
7. Deutsch, A.: *The Shame of the States*, Harcourt, Brace, New York, 1948.
8. Barton, W.E.: Advances in Administration in Psychiatry During the Past Fifty Years, A.W.R. ed., *Hope, Psychiatry's Commitment*, Brunner/Mazel, New York, 1970.
9. Barton, W., Farrell, M., McLaughlin, W., Lenehan, F.: *Impressions of European Psychiatry*, APA, Washington, D.C., 1958.
10. Barton, W.E., Barton, G.M.: *Mental Health Administration: Principles and Practices*, Human Sciences Press, New York, 1982.

INDEX